Ethical, Social and Legal DIMENSIONS OF SCREENING for Human Genetic Disease

Birth Defects: Original Article Series
THE NATIONAL FOUNDATION
March of Dimes

VOL. X, NO. 6
1974

Ethical, Social and Legal DIMENSIONS OF SCREENING for Human Genetic Disease

Editor
Daniel Bergsma, M.D.

Co-Editors
Marc Lappé, Ph.D.
Richard O. Roblin, Ph.D.
James M. Gustafson, Ph.D.

Assistant Editor
Natalie W. Paul

Genetics Research Group of the
Institute of Society, Ethics and the Life Sciences
Hastings-on-Hudson, New York

Symposia Specialists
MEDICAL BOOKS

STRATTON INTERCONTINENTAL MEDICAL BOOK CORPORATION
381 Park Avenue South, New York, New York 10016 and London

To enhance medical communications in the birth defects field, The National Foundation publishes the Birth Defects Atlas and Compendium, *an Original Article Series, Syndrome Identification, a Reprint Series and provides a series of films and related brochures.*

Further information can be obtained from:
Daniel Bergsma, M.D.
Vice President for Professional Education and
Director, Professional Education Department
The National Foundation-March of Dimes
1275 Mamaroneck Avenue
White Plains, New York 10605

Published by
Symposia Specialists
MIAMI, FLORIDA, 33161
Printed in the U.S.A.

Library of Congress
Catalog Card Number 74-78385
ISBN 0-88372-066-3

Received for publication January 29, 1974.

Contents

Introduction

In recent years, genetic screening has moved from relatively simple medical programs which are designed to alert individuals potentially affected by genetic disease to the need for treatment, to broader and more complex programs designed to detect and counsel individuals "at risk" for developing or transmitting genetic and genetic-related disease or disability. Among other factors, the advent of prenatal diagnosis for both simple and complex genetic disorders, combined with the possibility of selective abortion, and of carrier detection of prospective parents at risk for transmitting genetic disease have greatly increased the impetus for expanding screening programs. Prenatal diagnosis, which had been used almost exclusively where one or both parents were "at risk" as carriers of a serious genetic disease, could now be extended to mothers at risk for age-related disorders, particularly the Down syndrome, or to families with a history of neural tube defects. Some genetic screening programs already encompass markers indicative of future physiologic difficulties, such as $alpha_1$-antitrypsin (associated with emphysema) or adenosine deaminase deficiency (associated with combined immune deficiency) where there may be but vague prior indications of increased risk in the family.

The movement to cast the genetic screening net further and further afield has been hailed by some biomedical scientists as a welcome expansion of the health care services that society can bring to individuals and their families. Others have questioned the wisdom of the objectives of such programs and have perceived potential medical, psychologic and sociologic hazards in premature enlargement of the scope of extant genetic screening programs.

The papers in this series are the result of two years of deliberation, discussion and review among members of the Genetics Group of the Institute of Society, Ethics and the Life Sciences, Hastings-on-Hudson, N. Y., of the multifaceted problems posed by the advent of the technologic potential for mass genetic screening.* While no single group of papers can

---

*A preliminary publication of this Group's provisional findings appeared in the May 25, 1972, issue of the *New England Journal of Medicine (N. Eng. J. Med.,* *286*:1129-1132, 1972.)

meaningfully broach all of the issues generated by genetic screening, these papers are intended to begin a critical examination of some of its facets: its medical and philosophic underpinnings; its value premises; its operation, goals and effectiveness; and the prospects for its beneficial or deleterious impact on society generally. They were written with the conviction that society will require a heightened sensitivity to the ethical, legal and social questions posed by the rapid influx of genetic knowledge. Once screening moves away from the simple medical model of one-variant-gene/one-metabolic-abnormality to embrace a spectrum of simple and complex diseases with varying degrees of genetic determination and susceptibility to treatment, it will undoubtedly encounter a welter of novel medicolegal, ethical and social problems. Moreover, research screening where the objective is simply to uncover sufficient knowledge to understand the prevalence, etiology and pathogenesis of genetic-based human disease, itself poses major problems in the acquisition, interpretation and application of the genetic and medical knowledge which are the prerequisites to the understanding and control of human disability. Ideally, the papers in this series will add to the understanding and appreciation of the nonmedical as well as the medical parameters which go into assessing the large-scale impact of genetic screening in our increasingly technologic society.

Marc Lappé, Ph.D.
Program Director in Genetics
Institute of Society, Ethics
and the Life Sciences
Hastings-on-Hudson, N. Y.

All of these papers were prepared under an NIH Grant (No. RO 1 GM19922-01), made to the Institute of Society, Ethics and the Life Sciences.

Newborn Genetic Screening as a Concept in Health Care Delivery

A Critique

Marc Lappé, Ph. D. and Richard O. Roblin, Ph.D.

Introduction

The 1960s saw a dramatic increase in public interest in and legislative concern about genetic disease, which led to passage of state laws mandating newborn screening for phenylketonuria (PKU). Currently, 43 out of 50 states require PKU testing. Among these states, at least 18 have passed legislation which anticipates testing for other inborn errors of metabolism. The newborn screening laws in Kentucky and Maine, for example, authorize general testing of newborns for metabolic disease with the sole stipulation (in Maine) that the abnormality be expected to result in subsequent mental deficiencies. Thus, the legal basis for compulsory mass screening of newborns for genetic diseases other than PKU was established in several states as early as 1967. A legislative proposal which mandates an expanded newborn genetic screening program for six specific genetic diseases has recently been introduced in the New York State Legislature.* Since this proposal may augur a new wave of legislative activity in neonatal genetic screening, we believe it is important to review the rationale for such multiphasic testing programs.

The questionable justification of the early legislative activities to control PKU has been reviewed by Bessman and Swazey.[1] They concluded that "What we have done so far with PKU should give us no cause for

---

*New York State Senate bill S 7005.

Marc Lappé, Ph.D., *Associate for the Biological Sciences, Institute of Society, Ethics and the Life Sciences, Hastings-on-Hudson, N. Y. and* Richard O. Roblin, Ph.D., *Assistant Professor, Harvard Medical School, Infectious Disease Unit, Massachusetts General Hospital, Boston.*

pride or self-satisfaction. If we examine the situation in which we find ourselves, we may be able to construct a more intelligent and effective approach to the application of science to social questions." Others have noted that current screening tests have proliferated to some extent merely "because inborn errors of metabolism are a new and exciting group of diseases" and because the technology was available.[2] It is with these views in mind that we have written this paper. We will evaluate the prospects and desirability of expanded genetic screening programs in two parts: the first deals with the philosophic and political implications of genetic testing, the second with procedural and ethical questions.

Philosophic and Political Considerations in Screening for Disease

Implicit Value Assumptions in General Rationales for Screening

The World Health Organization (WHO) has defined medical screening as "the presumptive identification of unrecognized disease or defect by the application of tests, examinations, or other procedures which can be applied rapidly. Screening tests sort out apparently well persons who have a disease from those who probably do not."[3] Although this definition includes no explicit statement of the *ultimate* purpose of the screening process, the implied purpose is provision of health benefits to those who are found by screening. In the case of screening for genetic diseases, other objectives, such as the acquisition of scientific knowledge or provision of knowledge of genetic carrier status, can also be justified, but the stated purpose of screening is most often given as the detection of presymptomatic conditions in order to ameliorate or prevent later disease.[2]

The rationale for screening programs thus assumes that the benefits derived from treatment following early detection of disease will exceed those that would be possible if the detection were deferred. However, screening for *unrecognized* disease, as is usually the case in genetic screening, introduces novel medical, legal and moral aspects, since such screening conducts investigations which do not arise from a patient's request for advice on specific complaints. This led McKeown to conclude that such investigations should be considered "a presumptive undertaking, not merely that an abnormality will be identified if it is present, but that those affected will derive benefit from subsequent treatment or care."[4] If the diseases which are screened for are not amenable to treatment, there is some danger that screening may lead only to social and psychologic isolation of individuals without affording them direct health benefits. Isolation of detected, affected individuals is explicitly mentioned in a subsequent WHO definition which describes the objective of disease screening as the discovery, treatment and, if necessary, "isolation of individuals" who are suspected of "being a danger to their neighbors."[5] However, as one of us has previously emphasized,[6] the arguments for isolation of carriers of infectious agents do not apply in the case of carriers of deleterious genes.

Implicit Political Assumptions in Screening

While most current genetic screening programs identify existing but subclinical disease processes, some new programs (such as those which may be designed to detect adenosine deaminase deficiency and presumptive immune incompetence[7]) will identify *impending* disease or disability. These programs rest on the rationale that anticipation of disease is itself desirable because it allows identification of a population at high risk for later disability. The WHO definitions of screening fail to discuss the political implications of placing the health needs of individuals who are likely to develop disease at some time in the future above those who are currently suffering from disease (but who may be unable to seek or receive medical attention). For example, Wilson and Jungner state that "screening is an admirable method of combating disease, since it should help detect it in its early stages and enable it to be treated adequately before it obtains a firm hold on the community".[5] These authors note only in passing that screening may not be universally useful because of the prevalence of overt disease – but believe such disease is only a problem of developing countries. With the greater availability of money in developed countries, they believe "efforts can be made to extend the disease-free period of life by all possible means, including the detection and correction of early departures from normal health."[5]

Thus, while screening may have begun as a mechanism for detecting, isolating and treating the sick, it may in the future be directed more toward the identification and preservation of health. While this may appear but a minor shift in emphasis, it should not pass unnoticed, since "health" is generally the province of the affluent and sickness the province of the poor, even in developed countries. We believe that among the questions to be asked before a country begins to invest appreciably in mass genetic screening, is whether or not significant disability from overt disease has been reduced to the point where it is acceptable to mount major programs designed to prevent new genetic diseases. Mounting mass detection programs for genetic diseases whose incidence rates are very low, (ie less than 1 in 20,000), would probably reflect and encourage a restructuring of the philosophy of health care delivery away from one which has emphasized the aggregate good of reducing the societal impact of disease generally, and toward one which values maximization of individual health and well-being. The paper by Twiss in this series reviews some of the value aspects implicit in such a move.

Implicit Assumptions of Disease Causation

Genetic screening, in contrast to traditional disease screening, moves away from seeking individuals who have failed to adapt toward finding ones who are prone to fail to adapt. Since screening for genetic diseases has generally entailed looking for abnormal biochemical profiles which are assumed to reflect underlying genetic deficiencies, there is a tendency to assume that each genetic disease has a purely endogenous cause. This assumption is only partially true, since all genetic disabilities only become manifest after interaction with some environmental or metabolic component.

There may also be some tendency to think and act as if genetic diseases were exclusively caused by identifiable "bad genes." For example, Dent says, "This screening has become a new form of public health, in which local health officers . . . are having to reorient their thinking a little beyond the more usual search for bacteria or viruses, as they begin to seek out the abnormal genes."[8] However, experience with one of the best studied genetic diseases, PKU, has revealed that it is genetically heterogeneous[9] in that at least some biochemically deviant individuals are phenotypically normal.[10] Thus, there is some danger that a biochemical abnormality which is only a manifestation of normal genetic heterogeneity may initially be regarded as "deviant." This had led to inappropriate treatment with subsequent fatal consequences for a few individuals in the past.[8] Hopefully, consciousness of potential genetic heterogeneity will prevent recurrence of such tragedies.

One of the premises of adult multiphasic screening programs is that one is testing a population that has been subjected to an environmental "winnowing." Proponents of one concept of illness believe that much of adult ill health results primarily from the organism's failure or inability to ward off, adapt to, or compensate for environmental accidents and insults over time.[11] While acknowledging that in many instances there are underlying genetic predispositions to this inability, as in diabetes and perhaps hypertension, some would maintain that the principal causative agent in producing disease is the environment, not genetic predisposition. To the extent that this represents an accurate formulation, meaningful screening could only be done after environmental exposure; hence it is the childhood, adolescent or adult phenotype of the host which should receive the greatest attention in screening. An emphasis on the primacy of genetic factors would, of course, lead to the opposite conclusion. A middle path is clearly indicated since there is general agreement that the phenotype is defined by the interaction of genotype and environment (see the paper by Ehrman and Lappé in this series).

However, many components of the genotype may only be imperfectly visualized by the qualitative or quantitative assessment of gene products at birth, which themselves fluctuate after environmental exposure. On the other hand, if one wishes to *anticipate* genetic-based disease, neonatal screening may be the only opportunity to examine the organism before labile markers are disturbed through postnatal environmental interaction. Seen in this light, *the crux of the medical arguments for neonatal genetic screening is whether or not one can accurately predict the future sequelae of environmental exposure by a momentary look at the metabolic state of the newborn.* While this has proved true for some metabolic states (such as hyperphenylalanemia and likelihood of subsequent mental retardation), significant questions remain as to what other disordered metabolic states or genetic markers will be found to correlate strongly with disability later in life.

There is already evidence of statistical association between members of the HL-A group of human transplantation antigens and a number of diseases, such as celiac disease and chronic aggressive autoimmune hepatitis (HL-A 1 and 8), uveitis, Reiter disease and ankylosing spondylitis (W27), psoriasis (HL-A13, W17) and myasthenia gravis (HL-A 8 and possibly 1). (For example see Ref. 14.) Many other indices are discernible at birth which may or may not prove to have meaningful associations with later disease. These include protease inhibitors associated with alpha$_1$-antitrypsin deficiency which may predispose to chronic, obstructive lung disease (see the paper by Erbe in this series for a fuller treatment of this association), and alterations in immunoglobulin classes like IgA and IgE which may be associated with later atopy or allergic states. Obviously, before these associations are known with confidence, the decision to screen for such markers will rest on justifications other than the provision of immediate health benefits to the screened population.

When to Screen: Practical Examples of Programs Based on Different Disease-Causation Philosophies

Screening at birth for immunoglobulin (IgM), complement (C5), or enzyme (adenosine deaminase) deficencies[7,12,13] may be justified on the need to detect immunodeficiency diseases which predispose the individual in the future to the risk of neoplasia or serious bacterial infection. However, it is currently difficult to justify using HL-A haplotypes alone for ascertainment of disease risk.[cf 14] Such estimations are now based on weak statistical associations and the diseases themselves usually have strong environmental components, thereby reducing the imperative of newborn testing. However, we do suggest that it might be desirable that some screening efforts be directed toward individuals *after* they have been exposed to environmental "triggering" agents rather than before such exposure as would be the case in most immunodeficiency newborn screening.

For example, it has proved more beneficial for public health purposes to screen children for immune responsiveness *after* they have been exposed to natural infection or vaccination rather than before.[15] Mass screening for bacteriuria in the female population at risk for pyelonephritis may be more productive in school-age girls who have been exposed to bacterial infection than in younger, more immunologically naive subjects.[16] In both instances, a genetic determination of possible susceptibility to infection would likely have been unrevealing, since with the exception of adenosine deaminase deficency[13] or other rare genetic immune deficiency diseases, there are as yet few general correlates of genetic status at birth and susceptibility to infection.[cf12]

Procedural Considerations in Screening Programs for Genetic Disease

Current and Future Programs

To focus our discussion, we will consider three concrete examples of existing screening programs or technologies: first, screening for PKU; second, a hybrid program (in Massachusetts) which screens for PKU and several other metabolic abnormalities; and finally, new technologies which could lead to much broader screening programs.

PKU Screening. The most widespread neonatal genetic screening program in the United States is that for PKU. In PKU screening, one looks initially for infants with elevated (>2-4mg/100 ml) blood phenylalanine levels. Typically, PKU testing programs utilize a bacterial growth test devised by Dr. Robert Guthrie of the State University of New York at Buffalo.[17] Several drops of blood are taken from each newborn, dried on a filter paper disk and mailed to the testing laboratory. There, the disks are placed on a plate containing agar, bacteria and a specific bacterial inhibitory substance. The bacteria will grow only if a predetermined minimal concentration of phenylalanine (2 mg/100 ml) is present. If an increased zone of bacterial growth is observed on the test plate, the infant is *suspected* to have PKU.* The test has been automated to the extent that one technician can test on the order of 50,000 samples per year, and the cost of the materials per test is less than the 10 cent stamp required to mail the blood sample to the testing center. The major costs of the program are salaries, overhead and other equipment required to permit follow-up evaluation of those tentatively identified as having PKU.

The scientific assumptions which underly a mass screening approach to PKU detection and treatment have been outlined by Bessman and Swazey[1]: (1) The condition generally produces mental (and to some extent physical) retardation. (2) The cause of retardation is known (eg an accumulation of the substrate or one or more of its metabolites). (3) There exists a mass screening test which is not prohibitively expensive and which is reliable in the sense of being sensitive while yielding few false-positive or false-negative results. (There are also confirmatory diagnostic tests which can be used to verify presumptive positive results identified by the mass screening test.) (4) A special diet or other therapy started early enough and continued long enough will prevent retardation in individuals with the genetic defect. Bessman and Swazey have also pointed out the questions and problems involved in each of these assumptions.[1]

Since their analysis, additional cases of adults with serum phenylalanine levels above 14 mg/100 ml who are mentally "abnormal," but *not* retarded have been reported.[10] Progress has been made in distinguishing PKU from some other causes of hyperphenylalanemia in neonates,[9] but the existence of variants of classic PKU have, in Nitowsky's judgment, "made the diagnosis of PKU arbitrary."[18] He concludes further that, as of 1973:

1. Our knowledge of the natural history and variability of PKU is still incomplete.
2. The effectiveness of treatment of the disease (PKU) has not been accurately measured.

---

*Follow-up tests over a period of one to two months are required to confirm a diagnosis of PKU by distinguishing it from several other causes of high blood phenylalanine levels in the newborn.

3. We have inadequate information about the optimal age for institution of therapy, or levels of serum phenylalanine at which treatment should be undertaken, or the age at which treatment may be stopped.

Since PKU is one of the most intensively studied genetic diseases, Nitowsky's conclusions apply with even greater force to all other genetic diseases for which one might screen in the newborn period. (See the paper by Powledge for further analysis of Nitowsky.)

Hybrid Screening (PKU plus other metabolic disorders). Although most states currently test only for PKU, Massachusetts is evaluating a screening program for metabolic disorders which can detect about 30 different genetic abnormalities in the newborn.[19] Some aspects of the ten most frequent disorders are shown in Table 1.

The Massachusetts program uses three separate tests: (1) an umbilical cord blood sample taken at birth to screen for potentially lethal diseases like galactosemia where the earliest possible detection is vital, (2) a

Table 1. Metabolic Disorders and their Estimated Frequency among Newborn Infants in Massachusetts*

Disorder	*Total Screened*	*Total Detected*	*Frequency*	*Treatment Available*
†Phenylketonuria	981,361	67	1:15,000	Yes (dietary)
††Atypical phenylketonuria	981,361	57	1:17,000	Not indicated?
Iminoglycinuria	332,143	34	1:10,000	Not indicated
††Cystinuria (several types)	332,143	21	1:16,000	Yes
Hartnup disease	332,143	18	1:18,000	Yes, and biochemical disorder may resolve spont neously in adulthood?
Histidinemia	332,143	18	1:18,000	No, dietary restric not effective?
†Galactosemia	550,000	5	1:110,000	Yes
†Maple syrup urine disease	842,004	5	1:170,000	Yes (dietary, restriction of leucine, isoleucine and valine)
†Argininosuccinic acidemia	332,143	5	1:70,000	Yes (dietary, protein restriction)
Cystathioninemia	332,143	3	1:110,000	
†Homocystinuria	449,619	3	1:150,000	Yes in some cases

*Modified from reference 19.

†Disorders with definite clinical complications.

††Disorders that may or may not be associated with clinical disease.

peripheral blood sample taken soon after dietary protein has been introduced (usually two to four days after birth), and (3) urine samples taken when the newborn is 3-4 weeks old. The utility of this last approach is underscored by the fact that separation and identification of compounds in urine by paper chromatography has identified several "abnormalities" which would be missed if only the blood were examined. The "extra" testing is required to establish the significance of any "abnormal" result by eliminating false-positive results due for example to bacterial contamination or transient neonatal findings. At least three consecutive abnormal specimens are required to indicate a metabolic disorder requiring further investigation.

In its current form, the Massachusetts program screens 75,000 to 80,000 infants per year and detects 30-35 infants with some metabolic disorder, of whom about 60% subsequently manifest clinically significant disease.[19] The Massachusetts program costs the laboratory about $200,000 per year, or about $2.50 per infant screened. About 80% of the program's annual budget comes from a federal grant (U.S. Public Health Service); the remaining 20% comes from the Massachusetts Department of Public Health.

Multiphasic Genetic Testing. Although the Massachusetts Metabolic Disorder Screening Program is properly described as "multiphasic" in the sense of testing one sample simultaneously for several abnormalities of amino acid metabolism, it does not embrace the full spectrum of test possibilities. Recent developments in separation technology now make it possible to separate, identify and quantitate 20-25% of the several thousand biochemical components of the human organism. A group of Scandanavian scientists (Jellum, Stokke, and Eldjarn)[20-22] has used a combination of eight different gas-liquid chromatographic systems to detect 500 to 1000 different compounds in blood or tissue samples. Pauling and his associates have accomplished similar technical feats on human breath and urine vapor.[23] The Scandinavian workers have compiled a computerized library of the mass spectral analyses of 17,000 different compounds to facilitate identification of unknown specimens obtained. In a preliminary study of some 800 subjects these chromatographic technics led to the discovery of four entirely new metabolic disorders.[20] To date, approximately 40 new inborn metabolic abnormalities have been detected, many of them of clinical significance.*[22]

---

*It should be noted, however, that multiphasic biochemical testing by gas chromatographic systems promises to be considerably more expensive, both in terms of the cost of each individual test, and in terms of the follow-up tests required to evaluate the significance of any abnormal results obtained.

However, the question of the desirability of routinely applying such truly multiphasic testing to newborns remains largely unasked.

An exception is Reimendal and Sjovall,[24] who have utilized gas chromatographic technics for automated analysis of steroids in the blood, urine, tissues and feces. Since disorders of steroid metabolism (such as adrenogenital hyperplasia) are a significant component of neonatal genetic disease, they believe these and related steroid analysis technics might profitably be applied in appropriate populations of newborns.

Recent technical developments in biomedical engineering are beginning to make mass multiphasic testing appear more feasible. Automated tests are available to detect at least seven significant metabolic disorders: PKU, maple syrup urine disease, homocystinuria, histidinemia, valinemia, galactosemia and argininosuccinic aciduria.[17] While current tests rely on bacterial growth-facilitation assays of the Guthrie type, other developments which would permit greater ease of automation are on the horizon. For example, Ganger has described an apparatus with operating costs of about $5 per sample which will separate 11-13 amino acids from urine and 9-10 from serum in about 45 minutes.[25]

Gas chromatography,[26] centrichromatography[27] and thin-layer chromatography[28] coupled with computer diagnosis have made feasible quantitative analysis of biologically important compounds at the nanogram (10^{-9} gms) level. The use of stable, nonradioactive isotopes promises to permit a safe and quantitative means of screening follow-up for rare disorders. For example, nonradioactive amino acids can be used in conjunction with gas chromatography and mass spectrometry to define a number of disorders of leucine and tyrosine metabolism,[29] eg ketotic hyperglycinemia, sweaty feet syndrome and maple syrup urine disease.[cf 30] In view of the recent demonstration of an apparently effective dietary treatment of the "sweaty feet syndrome,"[31] as well as past demonstrations of the benefits of early dietary interventions for other branched-chain aminoacidurias,[30] this may prove an extremely valuable technic.

Establishing a Screening Program

At what point does one know enough about the natural history and variability of a given genetic disease to justify a mass screening program? It would be fruitful to answer this question using concrete examples since the consequences of the disease, efficacy and potential side-effects of current therapy, and sensitivity of screening tests vary for different genetic diseases. In addition, because most genetic diseases are so rare, large-scale screening programs may be required to identify a sufficient number of cases to permit assessment of genetic heterogeneity and efficacy of different therapies. In the face of these observations, we have concluded that neonatal screening programs for genetic disease might profitably follow a two-stage development.

During the first stage, pilot research screening programs whose goals are case finding and assessing variability of the disease (eg genetic heterogeneity) and the efficacy of proposed treatments would be appropriate. Safeguards appropriate to such research programs, such as insistence on informed consent, would be required during this stage (see paper by Fletcher, Roblin and Powledge in this series). A potential candidate for such a program would be testing for alpha thalassemia, where the clinical features of the carrier status have yet to be elucidated.[32]

After a pilot program had been in operation for some years and experience with disease variability and efficacy of treatment had been accumulated, the entire experience with the disease should be reviewed and a decision made about transition to the second stage, that of mass screening programs which aim to provide an established medical service to the entire population at risk. The archetypal second-stage program is represented by thalassemia trait screening, where inexpensive, automated technics have been perfected for rapid discrimination of this trait from iron deficiency and beta thalassemia.[33-36]

The current Massachusetts Metabolic Diseases Screening Program illustrates the emerging tendency to combine screening for PKU with simultaneous screening for other genetic diseases.[19,37] As rapid, inexpensive tests for diseases other than PKU are developed, there is a tendency to employ them in screening programs *without* careful analysis of whether the circumstances of the disease in question justify such screening. Guthrie, for example, has generally relied on an economic rationale to encourage multiple testing.[17] (We will deal with cost-effectiveness calculations in neonatal genetic screening in more detail below.) At this time, we simply note that lumping together neonatal screening for PKU (which could appropriately be considered a *service* program) and other genetic diseases for which screening is still in the *research* stage, blurs the distinction between them and may deny patient-subjects the safeguards to which they are entitled.

Current mass screening programs are limited in that they detect abnormal serum or urine concentrations of only a small number of specific biochemicals, usually amino acids. The multiple gas chromatographic or other automated systems referred to above[20-22,25-28] are capable of simultaneously measuring the concentration of *hundreds* of the biochemical compounds in human urine or breath. Such systems might be thought to represent the potential ultimate program in screening for neonatal genetic disease, and in modified form have come into increasing use.[cf 38] They are at least the ultimate in economic terms of "the maximum number of tests for your dollar." However, we believe such multiphasic systems will not prove useful for genetic screening until (1) extensive correlations are developed between "abnormal" levels of well-characterized biochemical compounds and clinical disease, and (2) the many other possible causes of abnormal concentrations (organic disease, changes in diet, slowly maturing neonatal enzyme systems) are excluded and the condition itself is proved to be of genetic origin.

As we have stressed, the validity of such screening systems rests on the assumption that the biochemical composition of the body fluids of the newborn will be an accurate index of the present and future health of the individual. This is an unproven assumption since it has yet to be determined how many of the biochemical substances which can be quantitated in the newborn will accurately reflect its adult functional genotype. For example, there is a question of which substances are its own gene products; some like alpha$_1$-antitrypsin globulin, may represent substances of maternal origin which have crossed the placenta. Another question remains regarding the permanence of structural gene products: some may be regulatory substances which are part of the early developmental needs of the fetus. We thus agree with the Scandinavian developers of these systems when they state: "It is our experience that computer techniques should mainly be applied on carefully selected patients rather than for screening large groups of patients."[21]

Research Potential of Newborn Screening

Several researchers have emphasized that the current value of multiphasic screening programs lies in their research potential. For example, Guthrie[17] has stated that multiphasic screening now "has enough scientific value to encourage mass screening for as many biochemical anomalies as possible. . . ." However, he qualifies his recommendation by noting that this is "always assuming that this can be done without dipping into funds needed for more urgent aspects of health care." Guthrie does believe that the ancillary research values of carefully designed screening programs will continually keep the balance of costs in favor of multiphasic screening. As long as screening procedures for the same cost "yield steadily increasing 'fringe benefits' of data on both pathologic and benign metabolic differences," he feels they will be justified. In a similar vein, Nitowsky has written:

Although the primary role of screening would appear to be preventive, there are other desirable objectives which continue to provide the major stimulus for development and use of these programs in the community. Screening permits early detection of poorly understood diseases and provides an opportunity to study them and to elucidate their pathophysiology.[18]

Hecker has also advocated prospective research objectives.[39]

The need for more data on the incidence, etiology and pathology of metabolic disease per se is often given as a sufficient rationale for mass screening. For example, Stern[40] has proposed that "pilot schemes in which all or a large random sample of newborn babies are screened for one or more inborn errors of metabolism" would be a good way to accumulate the necessary data. Although ethical questions are raised by any procedure which requires proxy consent for a nontherapeutic intervention, Hill and his colleagues believe such screening can be justified because it will stimulate investigation of just those metabolic pathways necessary for developing potential methodologies of treatment for detected infants.[41] We have previously stated that such research values are enhanced when they are linked to counseling or public health benefits.[6]

Organization of Neonatal Genetic Screening Programs

The economics of mass screening strongly favor the establishment of central testing centers, each of which might process 50,000 to 100,000 samples per year. As noted above, because of the low cost of the testing materials themselves, the major costs of starting each testing center are salaries, overhead and equipment. As a result, the cost per test for PKU decreases almost linearly up to 30,000 tests per year. Once each center does at least 30,000 tests per year, the cost *per test* decreases up to about 200,000 tests per year (H. L. Levy, personal communication). Thus maximization of overall cost-effectiveness for PKU screening programs would involve establishing 20-30 testing centers throughout the United States. Since PKU testing is currently organized separately by each state, this has led to suggestions that regional testing centers would be advantageous for those sections of the country where there are states with less than 30,000 newborn infants per year. Attempts to establish regional testing centers would raise legal questions, however, since public health legislation is an area traditionally left up to the individual states. (See the paper by Green and Capron in this series.)

Even now where one central testing facility serves an entire state, problems may exist in communication of positive results to parents of infants with PKU and their doctors and in appropriate follow-up. There are at least two potential sources of difficulty. First, because of the geographic separation of the testing center and the patient's location, effecting the repeated testing and follow-up required to unambiguously establish the PKU diagnosis will be more laborious and time-consuming. Treatment poses similar problems since "clinical experience has demonstrated that individual requirements for phenylalanine among PKU patients vary greatly,[cf8] [and] one child may require 3 times as much dietary phenylalanine as another to maintain the same blood level [of phenylalanine]."[17] Thus, periodic monitoring of the effects of the low phenylalanine diet is an essential component of the care of phenylketonurics. Many local medical facilities may lack the necessary equipment to do this periodic monitoring. Second, if genetic counseling of the parents is viewed as an essential component of the neonatal genetic screening program (as we believe it should be), delivering this health care component will require either visits by parents of PKU infants to the central testing and counseling center, or a "roving" genetic counselor.

The organization of neonatal genetic screening programs is intimately connected to the source of the funds for testing programs. To date, although state governments have shown themselves willing to mandate PKU testing, they are less willing to appropriate adequate funds to finance the screening programs. For example, the above cited Massachusetts Metabolic Disorder Screening Program receives only about 20% of its annual budget from the Massachusetts Department of Public Health. Without the federal grant which covers the remaining 80% of its costs, the Massachusetts screening program could not continue (H. Levy, personal communications). If the Massachusetts situation is typical, state legislatures have yet to face the true costs of neonatal genetic screening programs for PKU. Given the present funding pinch for most state legislatures, it may prove difficult to induce them to increase their appropriations for neonatal genetic screening programs. If federal funds continue to take up the slack in paying for genetic screening programs, one must ask whether there is an equal distribution of such funds so that all neonates share equally in the benefits from PKU diagnosis and treatment, and whether other medical priorities have been considered.

Cost-Effectiveness and Priorities in Neonatal Screening Programs

Many evaluations of neonatal genetic screening programs, including this one, are permeated by references to their "cost-effectiveness."

Following Pole,[42] we distinguish between cost-benefit analyses, which assess problems of *priorities*, and cost-effectiveness analyses, which evaluate different technics as solutions to a given problem. The problem of where genetic disease prevention and treatment stand in the scheme of national health *priorities* is an important one to which we have already alluded, but it is too complex for us to deal with in depth here. Instead, we advance a preliminary analysis of the problem of priorities among the different genetic diseases for which one might screen, as well as some consideration of the cost-effectiveness of PKU screening.

We assume that government funds for genetic disease screening and treatment will always be limited, and therefore the problem of which genetic diseases one should screen for will remain acute. If this is so, which parameters should be considered in establishing priorities among the many different genetic diseases for which we currently have the technologic ability to screen? We suggest that the following factors merit consideration: (1) the frequency of the genetic disease, (2) the severity as measured by impact on health and suffering (for examples see paper by Gustafson in this series), (3) its potential consequences if undetected and untreated, (4) the efficacy of currently available therapies, and (5) the *total cost* of a program which would test and treat all those neonates who are equally at risk for the disease. Four very similar parameters have been advanced independently by Shine and Lal.[43]

The frequency of different genetic diseases in the general population is relatively easy to measure through pilot screening programs. Relying on frequency data as the principal criteria has a strong appeal, since it can be measured objectively and can be known with some certainty.[44] Giving first priority to those diseases which are most frequent also appeals to our rationality, since it in some way promises to maximize the use of our scarce resources by attacking the most "widespread" problems first. However, the selection of frequency as a factor carries with it some important value assumptions. It suggests that we value maximization of the number of cases detected over equal treatment for all those at risk for genetic disease. Should not the consequences of leaving *any* individual with an aminoaciduria untreated also be considered? If general federal tax revenues are used to support neonatal genetic screening programs, do not potential cases of maple syrup urine disease and PKU have an equal claim on the common resources, even though PKU is approximately ten times more frequent?

Using some measurement of the severity of the potential consequences of different genetic diseases as a factor satisfies a common sense feeling that we ought to pay more attention to diseases which are life-threatening than to those which are merely incapacitating to varying degrees. However, there are difficulties which prevent straightforward application of the notion of severity to an assessment of genetic screening programs, as Gustafson extensively discusses in his paper in this series. First and foremost, assessment of the severity of different genetic diseases is a subjective judgment, one which may not be expressible in quantitative terms. Which is more "severe," living for 50 years in a mentally retarded state, or premature death within the first two weeks after birth? Even assuming it were possible to rank all the genetic diseases for which one can screen in terms of their severity by successive pair-wise comparisons, whose ranking would we accept as definitive for the purposes of allocating public funds?

We advanced "the efficacy of currently available therapies" as a factor because of our fundamental assumption that "if you can't treat it, don't screen for it" (except for purely research purposes). There are also considerable difficulties in assigning quantitative weight to the efficacy of available therapies for different genetic diseases. Which is more "efficacious," dietary therapy for galactosemia which can prevent the premature death, cataracts, liver and kidney disorders but perhaps not mental retardation, or penicillamine therapy which can reduce the chances of renal stones in cystinuria? How much more efficacious is one than the other? It is often impossible to assess efficacy of current therapies unambiguously, given the fact that published reports from different research groups seldom agree exactly on this point.[cf 30]

As a final factor we suggest estimation of the total cost of a neonatal screening program which would test *all* those neonates equally at risk for a class of genetic diseases, according to some classification scheme similar to that presented by Frimpter.[30] Compared with two of our other parameters, cost at least has the advantage of being calculable. But which elements of a screening program should be included in a calculation of its costs? All would probably agree to inclusion of the testing cost, but what about the cost of follow-up tests to definitively establish the diagnosis? Should the costs of treatment of the affected neonates and genetic counseling for their parents be included? Again, who should decide these questions?

Finally, assuming that our society were able to agree on some mechanism for ranking severity of different genetic diseases and assessing the efficacy of different available therapies, should all these factors count equally in reaching an overall priority rating for the different genetic diseases? Or, are there overriding values, hidden in our factors, that would compel us to give preference to one of the factors? Consider, for example, the fact that untreated galactosemia causes death within a few weeks after birth. Yet it is an extraordinarily rare condition.[37] There are neonatal screening tests which can detect galactosemia and a dietary therapy which prevents death (although it may not restore the galactosemic to perfect "normalcy"). Is not the value of life itself one of such supreme importance that it merits extra weight in the factor calculation of priorities, or is the rarity of the disease sufficient to disqualify its detection and treatment on the basis of distributory justice and scarce medical resources, as some have suggested.[43,45]

We have only attempted a preliminary analysis of the problem of establishing priorities among different genetic diseases and are conscious of having raised more questions than we have answered. However, we believe that, in the long run, we will be better served by grappling with the problems we have raised here than by resorting to arbitrary, simplifying assumptions such as lower limits on disease frequency for which screening is "reasonable."[43]

One assessment of the cost-effectiveness of PKU screening programs has been given recently by Guthrie[17]:

> The detection and treatment of one case of PKU represents an outlay (assuming it is the result of 10,000 such screening tests, each costing \$.50-\$4.00 in the U.S.) of up to \$50,000; but failure to detect that case means a child that must almost certainly be institutionalized for the rest of its life, representing an outlay of at least \$250,000 (average life span of 50 years, annual expenditure for custodial care \$5,000). The \$250,000 figure includes no allowance for the future earnings of the treated case, or of the tax income from such earning. The economics of mass screening will continue to rest, as they do now, on the demonstrated fact that prevention is cheaper than nonprevention.

In this calculation, the "costs" of the "technics" of either screening or not screening are compared. A more conventional cost-effectiveness calculation would compare two different technics of measuring serum phenylalanine concentrations, for example, comparison of the Guthrie tests with column chromatography.[28]

As noted above, there is a great need to establish which elements of the genetic screening program to include in the cost calculation. Clow and her colleagues in Canada[46] have made considerable progress in elucidating the parameters that go into a "total care" concept for dealing with genetic disease. We agree with Guthrie that the cost of treatment of PKU infants should be included in calculating the cost of the screening program. In addition, some provision should be made for long-term follow-up of female neonates with PKU, since they are quite likely to bear mentally retarded offspring unless treated with a special diet during pregnancy.[9] Finally, we believe that the cost of genetic counseling for the parents of neonates with PKU should be considered as part of the cost of a neonatal genetic screening program. These additional elements should especially be made part of screening programs where screening is made mandatory by law.

Priorities and Potential Values of Newborn Genetic Screening

It is evident from this discussion that medical priorities for multiphasic screening of newborns for their genetic composition are based as much on philosophy of disease as they are on the philosophy one attaches to screening itself. A decision to screen newborns with a battery of tests designed to discern the metabolic status (and hence approximate genotype) of every newborn through mass utilization of automated data gathering technics ultimately involves medical, social and political decisions. These decisions in turn will be based on the valuation we make of the health needs of our population and the conceptualizations we make in defining disability and well-being. Neonatal genetic testing, in contrast to adult testing, is now conceived of as a series of programs to detect those relatively few individuals who have severe metabolic disabilities (ie ones which are manifest at birth or shortly thereafter) for which specific therapies are possible. Included in this net, however, will be a much larger group of infants with metabolic abnormalities, eg tyrosinemia or hemoglobin Barts, which may be transient or clinically ambiguous conditions of *unknown* medical significance. While such data may be of inestimable research value, their gathering raises knotty questions of medical priorities. Increasing the size of the genetic screening net poses problems of potential stigmatization through societal response to uncovered genetic deviancy of unknown significance. Ultimately, multiphasic genetic screening must face the question of whether or not we should collect data about which we do not now know enough to act, but which may be crucial for effective intervention in the future. We believe that *medical priorities* will dictate that future screening programs embrace a wide spectrum of metabolic states of potential medical significance other than those strictly associated with genetic disease. The decision to screen or not to screen any population for multiple biochemical variants will in turn be based on a resolution of the value of such screening for realizing the health objectives of the society. Where there is appreciable disability from nongenetic diseases, prescriptive genetic screening will be less justified than where such disability has already been minimized. We agree with Buist and Jhaveri that "we should strive for methods aimed at solving common medical problems in addition to having tests for rare and esoteric disorders,"[2] but we would put particular emphasis on solving the "common" problems first.

We believe that the validity of newborn mass genetic screening hinges on the prospects of realizing true health benefits from its operation for a *significant* number of people. Since it is increasingly argued that the rarity of individual genetic disorders (singly and in aggregate) may *not* constitute a sufficient health burden compared to other health needs of the populace,[43] the justification for screening may well depend on its ancillary values. The following arguments can be made for expanding current programs of genetic screening:

1. Expanding screening to include testing for multiple biochemical markers of genetic and polygenic disease. Ideally such programs would allow the identification of a large number of individuals who are at risk for disease or disability directly or indirectly related to their genetic make-up. Genetic information taken at birth could provide critical *prospective* data for anticipating disease states. For example, comprehensive HL-A typing of transplantation antigens at birth could provide a means for determining the role of genetic factors in the etiology of a variety of conditions (eg ankylosing spondylitis or psoriasis).

The results obtained in any such screening program would allow population norms to be established for detecting medically important deviancy and would thus help in assessing the prospective health status of individuals. Such data would also provide statistical information against which deviant results on a population-wide scale could be better weighed than is now possible for most rare biochemical disorders. Some of the hemoglobin screening programs have already been expanded to encompass some of these objectives.[47,48] However, we would generally construe all programs of this type as "research screening" and consequently we would urge strict controls for ensuring confidentiality of data and for obtaining informed consent.

2. *Development and expansion of case-finding technics and treatment facilities to include the maximum number of genetic diseases now amenable to therapy.* We believe there are strong moral imperatives for this action, especially since only a portion of the 67 disorders now subject to treatment are currently objects of mass screening.[46] Motulsky, however, has urged that if such expanded testing for genetic diseases is to be done, it

must be based on a "careful assessment of the total effectiveness of such multi-disease programs."[44] We concur, and would emphasize the critical importance of cost-benefit analyses which incorporate some of the nonfinancial items alluded to above, and by others in this series.

3. *Add research-directed objectives to existing programs.* There are unusually broad research opportunities in mass genetic screening. Both the extraordinary amount of easily obtained data and the possibility of performing a variety of *prospective* studies, not otherwise possible, have frequently been cited. For example, an unselected population of neonates could be used to assemble base-line genetic data that would not only allow more precise determinations of the frequency of neonatal disorders or variants of disease, but would permit more precise correlations to be made between genetic, biochemical or chromosomal status at birth and subsequent medical history (see paper by Mellman in this series). Some of the unanticipated problems of such programs might include the difficulty of obtaining meaningful informed consent for multiple testing, the need for protecting confidentiality and the possibility of premature use of such data.

Ultimately, neonatal genetic screening rests on the philosophic assumption that it is the *genotype* which has paramount importance in determining fitness (in the non-Darwinian sense). This assumption is probably the topic of greatest intellectual controversy of our age; how it is to be resolved remains to be determined.

We believe it would be an error to regard neonatal genetic testing in isolation, or as an end in itself. To be effective and to function as part of the health care delivery system, screening must be closely coordinated with both diagnostic follow-up and treatment. As a U.S. Public Health Service spokesman declared, "Granted that screening, in case finding, is the first step; unless, however, it is part of a program that makes provision for diagnosis follow-up and treatment, screening itself loses all of its potential value."[49] Or, as Allan Chase has observed, unless the technical readiness for screening is developed synchronously with the medical readiness to act on all of the adverse health indices that are uncovered, "the research gains of such activities may well be offset by the human consequences of mass testing."[50]

References

1. Bessman, P. S. and Swazey, J. P.: PKU: A study of biomedical legislation. In Mendelsohn, E., Swazey, J. P., and Traviss, I. (eds.): *Human Aspects of Biomedical Innovation.* Cambridge:Harvard University Press, 1971.

2. Buist, N. R. M. and Jhaveri, B. N.: A guide to screening newborn infants for inborn errors of metabolism. *J. Pediat. 82*:511-522, 1973.
3. Commission on Chronic Illness in the United States: *Prevention of Chronic Illness.* Cambridge:Harvard University Press, 1957, vol. 1, p. 45.
4. McKeown, T.: Validation of screening procedures. In *Screening in Medical Care: Reviewing the Evidence.* New York:Oxford University Press, 1968, pp. 1-13.
5. Wilson, J. M. G. and Jungner, G.: Principles of screening for disease. *Public Health Papers,* No. 34. Geneva:WHO, 1968.
6. Lappé, M.: Human genetics. *Ann. N. Y. Acad. Sci., 216*:152-159, 1973.
7. Giblett, E. R., Anderson, J. E., Cohen, F. et al: Adenosine-deaminase deficiency in two patients with severely impaired cellular immunity. *Lancet, 2*:1067-1069, 1972.
8. Dent, C. E.: Preface – Other biochemical abnormalities. In Cusworth, D. C. (ed.): *Biochemical Screening in Relation to Mental Retardation.* New York: Pergamon Press, 1971, pp. vii-viii.
9. Cunningham, G. C.: Phenylketonuria testing – its role in pediatrics and public health. *Clin. Lab. Sci., 2*:44-101, 1971.
10. Perry, T. L., Hansen, S., Tischler, B. et al: Unrecognized adult phenylketonuria. *New Eng. J. Med., 289*:395-398, 1973.
11. Strehler, B. L.: *Time, Cells and Aging.* New York:Academic Press, 1962, pp. 11-19 ff.
12. Moore, E. C. and Meuwissen, H. J.: Immunologic deficiency disease. Approach to diagnosis. *N. Y. State J. Med.,* Oct. 15, 1973, pp. 2437-2445.
13. Pollara, B., Pickering, R. J. and Meuwissen, H. J.: Combined immunodeficiency disease and adenosine deaminase deficiency, an inborn error of metabolism. *Pediat. Res., 7*:362, 1973.
14. Smith, C.: Some implications of HL-A and disease associations. *Lancet, 1*:450, 1974.
15. Gold, E., Ferrier, A., Hatch, M. H. et al: Immune status of children one to four years of age as determined by history and antibody measurement. *New Eng. J. Med., 289*:231-235, 1973.
16. Asscher, A. W., McLachlen, M. S. F., Jones, R. V. et al: Screening for asymptomatic urinary tract infection in school girls. *Lancet, 2*:1-4, 1973.
17. Guthrie, R.: Mass screening for genetic disease. *Hosp. Pract., 7*:93-100, 1972.
18. Nitowsky, H. M.: Prescriptive screening for inborn errors of metabolism: A critique. *Amer. J. Ment. Def., 77*:538-550, 1973.
19. Levy, H. L.: Newborn screening for metabolic disorders. *New Eng. J. Med., 288*:1299-1300, 1973.
20. Jellum, E., Stokke, O. and Eldjarn, L.: Application of gas chromatography, mass spectrometry and computer methods in clinical biochemistry. *Anal. Chem., 45*:1099-1106, 1973.
21. Jellum, E., Stokke, O. and Eldjarn, L.: Combined use of gas chromatography, mass spectrometry and computer in diagnosis and studies of metabolic disorders. *Clin. Chem., 18*:800-809, 1972.
22. Jellum, E., Stokke, O. and Eldjarn, L.: Screening for metabolic disorders using gas-liquid chromatography, mass spectroscopy, and computer technique. *Scand. J. Clin. Lab. Invest., 27*:273-285, 1971.
23. Pauling, L., Robinson, A. B., Teranishi, P. and Cary, P.: Quantitative analysis of urine vapor and breath by gas-liquid partition chromatography. *Proc. Nat. Acad. Sci. USA, 68*:2374-2376, 1971.

24. Reimendal, R. and Sjovall, J. B.: Computer evaluation of gas chromatographic mass spectrometric analyses of steroids from biological materials. *Anal. Chem., 45*:1083-1089, 1973.

25. Ganger, S.: Rapid screening of aminoacidurias. *Amer. J. Med. Technol., 37*:434-439, 1971.

26. Hardy, J. P. and Kerrin, S. L.: Rapid determination of twenty amino acids by gas chromatography. *Anal. Chem., 44*:1497-1498, 1972.

27. Karasek, F. W. and Rasmussen, P. W.: Separation and identification of multicomponent mixtures using centrichromatography mass spectrometry. *Anal. Chem., 44*:1488-1490, 1972.

28. Ersser, R. S. et al: Some simple and rapid thin-layer chromatographic methods for clinical purposes. *Biochem. J., 122*:35, 1971.

29. Curtis, H. C. C., Vollmin, J. A. and Baerlocher, K.: Study of metabolic pathways in vivo using stable isotopes. *Anal. Chem., 45*:1107-10, 1973.

30. Frimpter, G. W.: Aminoacidurias due to inherited disorders of metabolism. *New Eng. J. Med., 289*:835-841; 895-901, 1973.

31. Levy, H. L., Erickson, A. M., Lott, I. T. and Kurtz, D. J.: Isovaleric acidemia: Results of family study and dietary treatment. *Pediatrics, 52*:83-94, 1973.

32. Schmaier, A. H., Maurer, H. M., Johnston, C. L., and Scott, R. B.: Alpha thalassemia screening in neonates by mean corpuscular volume and mean corpuscular hemoglobin determination. *J. Pediat., 83*:794-797, 1973.

33. England, J. M. and Fraser, P. M.: Differentiation of iron deficiency from thalassemia trait by routine blood count. *Lancet, 1*:449-453, 1973.

34. Pearson, H. A., O'Brien, R. T. and McIntosh, S.: Screening for thalassemia trait by electronic measurement of mean corpuscular volume. *New Eng. J. Med., 288*:351-3, 1973.

35. Esen, G. J. F.: A simple screening procedure for beta thalassemia. *Afr. J. Med. Sci., 3*:223-229, 1972.

36. Schriver, H. C. and Srivastana, P. C.: Differentiation of thalassemia minor from iron deficiency. *Lancet, 2*:154-155, 1973.

37. Shih, V. E. et al: Galactosemia screening of newborns in Massachusetts. *New Eng. J. Med., 284*:753-758, 1971.

38. Raine, D. N., Cooke, J. R., Andrews, W. A. and Mahon, D. F.: Screening for inherited metabolic disease by plasma chromatography, (Scriver) in a large city. *Brit. Med. J., 3*:7-13, 1972.

39. Hecker, R.: The investigation of the patient: Modern developments including automated multiphasic health screening and the use of computers in medicine. *Med. J. Aust., 2*:492-496, 1972.

40. Stern, J.: Other biochemical abnormalities. In Cusworth, D. C. (ed.): *Biochemical Screening in Relation to Mental Retardation.* New York:Pergamon Press, 1971, pp. 9-21.

41. Hill, A. and Zaleski, W. A.: Screening for metabolic disorders associated with mental retardation. *Clin. Biochem.,* March 5, 1972, pp. 33-45.

42. Pole, J. D.: The cost-effectiveness of screening. *Proc. Roy. Soc. Med., 64*:1256-1257, 1971.

43. Shine, I. and Lal, S.: Need for screening as related to frequency of disease. *New Eng. J. Med., 289*:273, 1973.

44. Motulsky, A. G.: Need for screening as related to frequency of disease. *New Eng. J. Med., 289*:273, 1973.

45. Switkes, P. A., Gordon, J. B., Shih, V. E. and Levy, H. I.: Cost benefits of neonate screening. *New Eng. J. Med., 285*:239-40, 1971.
46. Clow, C. L., Fraser, F. C., Laberge, C. and Scriver, C. R.: On the application of knowledge to the patient with genetic disease. *Progr. Med. Genet., 9*:159-213, 1973.
47. Barnes, M. G. et al: A comprehensive screening program for hemoglobinopathies. *JAMA, 219*:701-705, 1972.
48. Garrick, M. D., Dembure, P. and Guthrie, R.: Sickle cell anemia and other hemoglobinopathies. *New Eng. J. Med., 288*:1265-1268, 1973.
49. Chase, A.: Cited in *The Biological Imperatives: Health, Politics, and Human Survival.* Baltimore:Penguin Books, 1971, p. 58.
50. Ibid p. 82.

Genetic Screening as a Political and Social Development

Tabitha M. Powledge, M.S.

In the past, society generally sought to control not a status or condition but an act . . . In the criminal realm, American society is increasingly restricting societal interference to situations of clear and present danger; the therapeutic trend, however, is to prevent such danger from arising through earlier societal intervention. Clearly, the more society departs from the old standard of the overt act and the more it permits the compulsory control of a vague condition of status, the more the doors to potential abuses of power and to assaults upon individual diversity are opened.[1]

What social or even medical utility is to be accorded diagnostic ability if it is not accompanied by effective action and an acceptable outcome?[2]

The object of screening for disease is to discover those among the apparently well who are in fact suffering from disease. They can then be placed under treatment and, if the disease is communicable, steps can be taken to prevent them from being a danger to their neighbours. In theory, therefore, screening is an admirable method of combating disease, since it should help detect it in its early stages and enable it to be treated adequately before it obtains a firm hold on the community.

In practice, there are snags.[3]

Introduction

The history of public health may have begun – as one chronicler[4] asserts – with Sumerian drains; but medical screening procedures are quite a recent chapter in that ancient history, and genetic screening is more recent yet. Medical screening is the outcome of many disparate motives

---

Tabitha M. Powledge, M.S., *Research Associate for Genetics, Institute of Society, Ethics and the Life Sciences, Hastings-on-Hudson, N. Y.*

and capabilities. Its chief aim, at least at the beginning, was the primary prevention of disease, and one of its chief motives was economic.[3] On the simplest level, as Pole[5] and others have pointed out, it saves the doctor's time.

The assembly line in medicine is, philosophically at least, a quintessentially democratic procedure. It seems to offer the same promise of population-wide distribution of the product (in this case, health), at the same comparatively low *per capita* cost, as the assembly line in Detroit. Thus it is probably not an accident that screening is undergoing serious criticism at this time; so are other assembly-line procedures, in medicine and elsewhere. Now that we have grown used to the benefits attendant on mass efforts, we are beginning to have leisure to notice the drawbacks.

Screening is also at the heart of the technology that has worked drastic changes in some areas of American medicine without concurrently redesigning the delivery system, which has in turn led to a good deal of agitation for improving that system. Such demands are not only coming from the radical fringes, but in such centrist journals as *Scientific American.* In its pages, William Glazier[6] recently urged that technology be used to solve delivery problems:

> The answer to the mismatch of technology and delivery is for medicine to orient itself toward a more interventionist approach, by which I mean that the physician and the medical system should be prepared to take the initiative to the patient. The system should reach out to people, seeking out those who for genetic reasons or because of their work or way of life may have a predisposition to a disease, carrying on health education among those at risk, pressing among the poor the case for better nutrition for children so as to forestall crippling disabilities in later life and reminding patients who are identifiably ill of the need for specific measures of treatment. . . . Preventive medicine was once a wholly public concern. . . . Now it has also become a private concern.

There is also a strain of argument against such mass procedures. Black and Riley[7] have recently urged that high priority be given to development of prostheses and diagnostic aids, and low priority to patient monitoring and population screening. They regard the latter as too costly and not very useful and state "that in making people too health conscious we increase the incidence of neurosis."

Screening: Background

Screening began in the early part of this century in an effort to control endemic communicable diseases such as malaria and syphilis, and achieved particular success with pulmonary tuberculosis. Interest in screening for chronic noncommunicable disease began only after the Second World War. The first large-scale population screen for diabetes, for instance, took place in 1947. Multiphasic screening, in which several different tests are run simultaneously, frequently on the same sample, was developed at about the same time, but was strongly endorsed by the American Public Health Association only in 1960.[3]

Wilson and Jungner[3] have pointed out that sociologic factors are critically important in the development of disease screening. Thus, when social conditions improve, communicable disease declines and chronic disease becomes more prominent. This is now the situation in industrialized countries, while developing nations still face massive problems with communicable disease.

The benefits of mass screening for communicable disease have been largely demonstrated, but the value of such screening for chronic disease is somewhat in doubt.[3] That may be one reason why genetic screening has been especially controversial. It does not seem to fall neatly into either category. Genetic disease is certainly chronic and usually degenerative. Yet it is also, in a very special sense, communicable.

However, there is a critical difference between the usual medical procedure, where the patient seeks the doctor's help, and screening, where the patient is actively sought by the doctor. Cochrane and Holland,[8] for instance, state the problem succinctly:

> We believe there is an ethical difference between everyday medical practice and screening. If the patient asks a medical practitioner for help, the doctor does the best he can. He is not responsible for defects in medical knowledge. If, however, the practitioner initiates screening procedures, he is in a very different situation. He should, in our view, have conclusive evidence that screening can alter the natural history of disease in a significant proportion of those screened.

Screening: Criteria

Since the early days of screening, there have been attempts to set up criteria. If the procedure under consideration fails to fulfill all the specified conditions, then it has been regarded by the group studying it as not acceptable. That has not, however, always meant that the procedure has been abandoned. On the contrary, the approach has been "screen now, validate later," which has meant that programs are instituted first and *then* evaluated (partly, of course, out of necessity; one cannot evaluate without numbers). It is obviously much more difficult to dismantle a going concern than to prevent one from getting started in the first place. Thus there are a surprising number of screening programs around – some of which have enthusiastic public support – which are not at all highly regarded among health professionals. Why they continue probably has something to do with vested interests of researchers, relatives and manufacturers of testing devices. But it may ultimately be the result of our terror of doing nothing when we could be doing something, even if that something is inadequate by rational criteria. And often, the alternative to screening *is* simply to do nothing. Powles[9] has pointed out that momentum based on past achievements is no doubt also responsible for enthusiasm for screening. He notes:

> Despite the evidence to the contrary, it is widely believed by both patients and their doctors that industrial populations owe their higher health standards to "scientific medicine," that such medical technology as currently exists is largely effective in coping with the tasks it faces and that it offers great promise for the future.

The criteria for screening have varied somewhat from study to study, but are generally drawn along similar lines. Among ten proffered by Wilson and Jungner,[3] for instance, are these: (1) The condition should be an important health problem (which might mean rare but serious, not just frequent). (2) There should be an accepted treatment ("Of all the criteria that a screening test should fulfill, the ability to treat the condition adequately, when discovered, is perhaps the most important"). (3) The cost of case finding should make sense in relation to medical expenditure as a whole.

In the mid-1960s, the Nuffield Provincial Hospitals Trust in Britain brought together a working party to study screening. That group hammered out criteria and then applied them to ten currently popular screening procedures, publishing the results in 1968. Only four passed their test. McKeown,[10] who chaired the group, pointed out that the screening must be effective and must also make better use of limited resources than other alternatives. Further, he declared:

> Except for research and the protection of public health . . . no one should be expected to submit to the inconvenience of investigation or the anxieties of case-finding without the prospect of medical benefit. The obligation exists even when the patient asks to be screened, for his request is then based on the belief that the procedure is of value, and if it is not, it is for medical people to make this known.

He also outlined three aims screening may properly have. First, it may be essentially a research project, with the same kind of ethical restrictions as other research projects. (A program in the process of validation might be regarded in this light, and would not necessarily have to fulfill the criteria at the outset.) Second, it may be a public health situation, for instance, the pursuit of a particular infectious disease presenting grave risk to society. (In this case perhaps all the criteria, particularly the economic ones, need not be rigidly met.) The working party established criteria for a third kind of screening program, called prescriptive screening, which seeks to make a contribution to the health of particular individuals. It is in this kind of screening that the criteria should be most carefully observed.

Genetic Screening: Criteria

The criteria have been applied to genetic screening for inborn errors of metabolism by Nitowsky.[11] For him, there are four standards: (1) The test must be easy and effective. (2) It must be oversensitive: some false positives are permissible, but false negatives are not. (3) There must be prompt study of all suspected positives to distinguish among variants. (4) There must be some treatment – or at least some kind of benefit for the patient.

This paper's thesis will be that the institution of medical procedures has social and political causes. It will examine genetic screening's brief history, in the process attempting to identify some of the conditions that have led to screening in the past and may do so again in the future. It should also become clear that genetic screening is in some ways very much like other kinds of screening, up to and including its failure to fulfill the proper criteria.

Genetic Screening

The Search for Disease

Genetic screening (here arbitrarily defined as the search for those suffering from or carrying a disorder of relatively simple inheritance) really began only about ten years ago, with large-scale testing of newborns for phenylketonuria (PKU). Adoption of this procedure as standard medical practice in most states has been extraordinarily rapid, despite a certain amount of professional disagreement over the proper methods of dealing with the disease.

Persons homozygous for PKU lack adequate phenylalanine hydroxylase activity. This enzyme is critical to proper metabolism of phenylalanine in the body. In ways not yet clearly understood, the condition leads to severe and irreversible intellectual deterioration. A diet low in phenylalanine instituted shortly after birth (which presents its own difficulties, since this amino acid is ubiquitous) is thought to prevent the worst consequences of the disorder, and is said to result in a child with an IQ in the normal range. Scattered reports on the diet – not all of them favorable – appeared in the literature in the late 1950s and early 1960s. The simple, inexpensive Guthrie screening test was introduced in 1963. Bessman and Swazey[12] have brilliantly demonstrated how these technics, imperfect as they were, were seized upon by several interested parties who, out of motives that were generally admirable, combined forces in a strong – and successful – campaign to institute newborn screening for PKU.

The first law specifying compulsory testing of newborns for PKU was passed in Massachusetts in 1963, but the state had instituted a voluntary program the year before. Within 18 months, 30 states had passed such laws; today 43 states mandate PKU screening for all newborns, and the remaining states screen voluntarily.

Although many of the arguments about PKU screening are technical and medical (and have been reviewed[11,13] often enough so that they will not be dealt with here), one argument has centered on the question of whether the screening should be compulsory or not. The stated justification for compulsion, of course, has been the desire for 100% coverage, felt to be unattainable with voluntary procedures. There are at least two available U. S. studies which permit some comparisons. Illinois passed a voluntary testing bill in 1963; a mandatory one was signed there two years later. Since 1966, more than 96% of Illinois newborns have been screened, compared with about 60% prior to the passage of the compulsory bill.[14] The state of Washington resisted a state law on PKU until 1967; in that year 69% of the state's newborns were screened under its voluntary program.[15] The authors felt this did not compare too badly with the 90% compliance one could reasonably expect under mandatory legislation. Although they believed that a mandatory law would probably have accelerated the screening somewhat, they also noted: "The importance given to the increase in screening efficiency has to be weighed against the problems in legislation of medical practice. There is no way to objectively measure the relative weight of these factors; it becomes a matter of opinion."

There is certainly no dearth of opinion. Nitowsky's[11] recent, comprehensive review of some of the technical problems endorsed screening (although not necessarily compulsion):

> I believe that we shall be forced to the conclusion that our knowledge of the natural history and variability of PKU is incomplete, that the effectiveness of treatment of the disease has not been accurately measured,

that we have inadequate information about the optimal age for institution of therapy, or the levels of serum phenylalanine (PA) at which treatment should be undertaken, or the age at which treatment may be stopped. Despite these unanswered questions, and the obvious lack of adequate validation of prescriptive screening, I do not believe we should turn backwards. Our intuition and empirical judgements would deter us from altering current practice.

Cunningham's[13] massive review makes a similar point. This probably represents the majority view. Bessman and Swazey[12] use the same data on the uncertainty of the PKU situation to argue strongly against the laws, and perhaps (although they are not quite so clear on this point) against the screening too. Thus, there is widespread agreement that there are grave problems with the PKU screening procedure; the disagreement arises in deciding how to proceed from there.

One point generally not emphasized in discussions of compulsory screening of all newborns for PKU is that, like many other genetic diseases, it is found in highest frequency in one population: in this case, people of northern European descent. Ethnic boundaries of this sort considerably weaken the argument for universal testing. In fact, Washington, D. C., grew so disenchanted with its PKU program that it abandoned it, according to *Medical World News* (November 19, 1971). Three years of testing the largely black newborn population there, at an annual cost of $100,000, had failed to turn up a single case.

It did not take long for PKU testing to expand to include testing of newborns for several other abnormalities, for technical and economic reasons. The movement was no doubt given a boost by a 1968 WHO report[16] on the state-of-the-art in screening for inborn errors of metabolism, even though its conclusion was somewhat equivocal: "The value of mass screening for certain diseases and in particular countries is beyond dispute. Its relevance to preventive medicine and its value in providing information about the human gene pool cannot be fully assessed at present." But by 1970, Scriver[17] estimated that 90% of live-born North American babies were being screened for one or more recessive metabolic disorders in government programs. The Massachusetts Metabolic Disorders Screening Program, for instance, screens about 90,000 newborns a year, spending $1.75 per infant, but is said to save the state more than a million dollars annually in lifetime custodial costs.[18] Several conditions besides PKU are screened for; about 1 in 2,500 newborns is found to have some metabolic abnormality, and 60% of these are clinically serious.[19] Even this program, which has screened almost a million babies, had some notable setbacks: a four-year hunt for galactosemia that screened 374,341 newborns (at a cost of 20c each) resulted in only one diagnosed and one presumptive case of these defects in galactose metabolism. Furthermore, both infants were dead before the results of their tests were known.[20] (In defense of the galactosemia program, it should be noted that prior European data had indicated many more cases would be found.) Then, in the spring of 1972, two more cases were discovered; at the time of the report[21] they were both on dietary therapy and clinically well. A British study[22] reported similar problems: two out of its four galactosemia cases died before the results were in. This group points out that likely benefits of newborn screening cannot be assessed until there are good data on incidence, but ends up recommending galactosemia screening only for sick infants, rather than all of them. This kind of argument is typical of lack of professional agreement on proper procedures, a continuing feature of genetic screening programs.

Most of these newborn tests are done on cord and peripheral blood; routine urine screening is also recommended.[23] (With these procedures, of course, many nongenetic conditions can also be detected.) Newborn sickle cell screening is being done in a few places; recent announcement[24] of a new test for hemoglobinopathies, using the same specimen as the PKU test, will no doubt make it more widespread. As this is being written, the New York State legislature is preparing to consider a bill that would add six more tests to its compulsory newborn testing program for PKU.* The conditions to be sought are sickle cell anemia (homozygote only), maple syrup urine disease, adenosine deaminase deficiency, homocystinuria, histidinemia and galactosemia. And this bill does not represent the first attempt to expand newborn genetic screening by law. Montana legislated expansion of its newborn screening in the spring of 1973.

There is certainly a host of problems inherent in expanded newborn testing, however. Birmingham, England, has been screening 20,000 newborns annually for 20 amino acid disorders, and has had to reorganize many of its services (pediatric, laboratory and so forth) as a result of the increased case load.[25] This kind of accessory difficulty is all too often not anticipated when program expansion is undertaken. The result is that the few positive cases that are identified don't get the kind of treatment the screen was designed to provide.

Clow et al,[26] participates in a large genetic screening network centered in Quebec, are emphatic about the expanded need for supportive services, once large-scale screening programs have been instituted. Their reported cost, $2.50 per infant, includes multiphasic mass screening, diagnosis,

*This bill is now law.

counseling and even treatment of those found to be affected, as well as pilot research projects and screening programs in high-risk groups. They estimate the potential North American case load of babies with PKU, histidinemia, cystinuria and maple syrup urine disease is about 675 in the first year of a screening program, rising to 3,375 in the fifth year. Their paper, a comprehensive description of an exceptional program, also provides interesting data on the question of compulsion. Participation in the program is completely voluntary; there is even a form of parental consent given, and yet more than 90% of the newborns are screened, a figure fully in line with compulsory programs in the United States. It took only about 18 months for the Canadians to achieve this degree of participation. The figures are similar for Ontario; its voluntary program reached 94.5% of newborns between 1966 and 1971.[27] One inescapable conclusion is that participation is clearly far more a function of desire, organization and the availability of testing facilities than of legal sanctions. It is conceivable that the voluntary programs in Washington and Illinois, previously cited, made a poorer showing than later compulsory programs there largely because they preceded them in time, and were thus hampered by lack of organization and available laboratories. In any case, the Canadian example provides a clear demonstration that a voluntary program can indeed achieve as much participation as one that is mandatory, and that is in itself a valuable lesson.

There have also been a number of projects to screen newborns for chromosome anomalies, but these are fairly clearly research efforts, rather than disease detection screens. Their aim has largely been to determine actual newborn incidence of chromosome defects. For instance, at least 13 surveys of newborns have looked for XYY infants.[28] Most newborn XYY individuals are being followed in prospective studies intended to confirm or disprove the reported association of the extra Y chromosome with sociopathic behavior. This kind of study, which seems quite clearly to fall into the research category rather than that of disease screening, presents unique ethical problems for the investigators, particularly on issues of disclosure.

The Search for the Carrier

Despite the fact that newborn metabolic screening may not fulfill all the usual criteria for screening, even when judged by its partisans, it at least represents attempts to find and treat disease. Thus it clearly falls into the traditional pattern that has historically justified screening programs.

The late 1960s, however, witnessed a movement toward a completely different kind of screening, aimed not at the diseased homozygote but at the carrier heterozygote; not just at the eradication of disease, but the eradication of babies with the disease. Kass[29] has asked,

> In the case of what other diseases does preventive medicine consist in the elimination of the patient-at-risk? Moreover, the very language used to discuss genetic disease leads us to the easy but wrong conclusion that the afflicted fetus or person *is* rather than *has* a disease. True, one is partly defined by his genotype, but only partly. A person is more than his disease. And yet we slide easily from the language of possession to the language of identity, from "He has hemophilia" to "He is a hemophiliac," from "She has diabetes" through "She is diabetic," from "The fetus has Down's syndrome" to "The fetus is a Down's." [Italics added.]

It can hardly be overstressed (because it has been so frequently ignored) that this movement represented a brand new step in screening, one that might legitimately be called the ultimate in preventive medicine.

To date, heterozygote screening in this country has concentrated largely on two diseases: Tay-Sachs and sickle cell anemia. Those diseases represent two different types of screening situations, and will certainly be prototypes for other programs that will inevitably develop in tandem with technology. (See the papers in this series by Kaback and Murray.)

Tay-Sachs disease is not common, even among the population where it is most frequent: Jews of eastern European ancestry. Since the carrier prevalence in this population is about 1/30, the newborn incidence is about 1/3,600 (1/30 × 1/30 × 1/4), compared with 1/360,000 in other populations. About 50 children with Tay-Sachs disease are born in this country every year; almost all are Ashkenazi Jews.[30] The progress of the disease has been described many times: how a happy, normal-appearing baby begins after a few months inexplicably to regress, then to degenerate, then dies before the age of five, blind, paralyzed, unresponsive. In addition to the personal devastation inflicted upon a family with a Tay-Sachs child, the disease's financial toll can be crushing. The complete care required in a child's last years can cost $40,000 annually – and the better the care, the longer the child will live. Hexosaminidase A, the enzyme whose absence causes such calamity, was identified in 1969; the first prenatal diagnosis, involving a test for the enzyme in cells cultured from amniotic fluid, was reported the following year. This makes possible diagnosis early enough for a safe abortion if the fetus turns out to be affected. A simple, inexpensive test to detect the less-than-normal hex A activity in a heterozygote also paved the way for large-scale carrier detection, among people who had no notion they were at risk because the disease had not yet made an appearance in their families.[30] Thus in Tay-Sachs carrier screening, an easily identifiable population is offered the chance to greatly lower the incidence of an irrevocably fatal disease and help assure the birth of unaffected children. It becomes very difficult to find telling arguments *against* screening in this situation. Any other course appears inhumane.

Sickle cell anemia is, of course, quite a different story. For one thing, it is a good deal more common. About 8% of American blacks born are heterozygotes; the estimated frequency of homozygotes is about 1/625 at birth and probably about 1/875 among the U. S. black population as a whole, due to mortality from the disease.[31] About 1,200 new cases a year are diagnosed.[32] But sickle cell trait is not uncommon in many non-black populations, such as southern Italians and Sicilians, northern Greeks, central and southern Indians and some Amerindians – in fact, almost any area of the world where falciparum malaria, against which it seems to offer some protection, is or was endemic. It is also found in American descendants of those populations[33] (though, of course, much less frequently than among blacks; the incidence of the trait among white populations has been estimated at 0.08%).[34] But at the outset, the population that can usefully be screened is not nearly so well defined as in Tay-Sachs. Screening has, nonetheless, concentrated on blacks.

While it has been estimated that half the children with sickle cell anemia die before they are 20,[32] many live twice that long and more; the disease is not invariably fatal. It is generally painful and debilitating, but patients are living longer and more useful lives as a result of improved treatment, which is likely to improve more in the not-too-distant future.

Further, screening tests commonly in use have not always been reliable, and there is not yet perfect agreement on the best laboratory methods.[35] Finally, prenatal diagnosis for this condition, while possibly on the way,[36] is not yet a reality, and will in any case not be widely available for some time. Thus carrier-carrier couples do not currently have the healthy-child option of Tay-Sachs couples unless they resort to adoption or artificial insemination with a noncarrier donor. Each of these alternatives is, of course, currently plagued with difficulties of its own. These characteristics – an ill-defined target population, a wide range of seriousness in the disease, and lack of prenatal diagnosis – combine to make the arguments for sickle cell screening much less compelling than they are for Tay-Sachs (although the ethicist Ramsey[37] and others have argued for such screening on grounds that it facilitates responsible parenthood if its aim is to prevent conception).

The genesis of sickle cell screening may have been the 1964 publication of a WHO technical report,[38] which contained a discussion of screening and public education programs in parts of Italy where thalassemia, a recessive hemoglobin disorder also known as Cooley anemia, is common. The Italian program was specifically aimed at discouraging carrier-carrier marriages, and the WHO report suggests: "The same measure could be readily applied to sickling and sickle-cell anaemia, and, if accepted by a high proportion of the population, could lead to a dramatic fall in sickle-cell anaemia in a single generation." The consequences of sickle cell screening in this country should make it very clear that standards suitable for a nation with a relatively homogeneous population, where divorce and abortion were both illegal and sinful, cannot necessarily be transferred intact across the Atlantic to a country with a variety of beliefs and colors, and a special set of political problems in the target population. It is time to point out once again – even though the truism will no doubt continue to be ignored – that culture plays a major role in the usefulness of any medical procedure, and should be taken into consideration in the planning stages of new programs.

The sickle cell argument has been considerably muddied by some data suggesting that heterozygotes can on occasion suffer ill effects (for instance, anoxia) as a result of their one gene for sickle hemoglobin. In 1970, Jones et al[39] published a report on the sudden, inexplicable deaths, after exercise at moderate altitude, of four young military recruits. The studies suggested that sickle cell trait, which the four had in common, was responsible. This resulted in some agitation for preinduction screening of blacks, and even a suggestion[40] that those with the trait be excluded from military service altogether. This would be a radical move, since the military has been one of the few avenues to the middle class easily available to American blacks, and such a measure would effectively exclude as many as 1 in 12 from that avenue. The National Academy of Sciences-National Research Council set up a committee to investigate. Its report[41] was issued in February 1973 and recommended that all recruits, regardless of race, be screened for S-hemoglobinopathies before undergoing basic training, and that certain limitations be placed on the tasks performed by sickle cell heterozygotes (for instance, they should not be allowed to pilot or copilot a plane). The study also concluded that data on pathology in the heterozygote were inadequate, and that further research (in the form of a prospective study of recruits screened in the next two years) would be necessary for a true assessment of possible risks. (On the other hand, a recent study[42] of black professional football players – surely our national exemplars of good health – revealed that 6.7% of them were sickle cell heterozygotes, a percentage not significantly different from the population-wide prevalence.) There is, however, the real possibility that an appreciable portion of an already deprived group might have to cope with this further accusation of inadequacy. The political and social consequences of this kind of research are unpredictable, but certainly potentially explosive.

Furthermore, if the sickle cell heterozygote is found to be at risk for physical problems, it is surely not a fantasy to predict that other heterozygotes may also fall into that category some day. At that point, carrier screening might legitimately fall within the boundaries of traditional screening, the search for disease, after all.

It has become increasingly clear that the arguments in favor of sickle cell screening have had more to do with politicians' desires to do something dramatic (and comparatively inexpensive) for a neglected population, and doctors' desires to encourage black interest in health in general, than with the medical wisdom of a current program of carrier screening per se.[43]

The major difference between screening for Tay-Sachs and for sickle cell, however, has been in the way the testing is organized. On the whole, the voluntary Tay-Sachs approach has been careful to enlist the support, enthusiasm, sponsorship and persuasive abilities of Jewish organizations, so that there appears to be a groundswell of demand for the testing. This kind of community participation has historically been important for screening.[44] There has furthermore been a good deal of emphasis on community education and involvement; in general, the Tay-Sachs programs give the impression of being thoughtful, careful and well organized. Furthermore, they are aimed at a group whose high socioeconomic status and educational level renders it exceptionally open to new medical ideas.[45] In a Tay-Sachs screening in Washington, D. C., for example, more than 46% of the participants had some postgraduate schooling.[46]

The contrast provided by the sickle cell situation is now well known: one clinician[47] has repeatedly called it a new sickle cell crisis. Problems of the programs have been reviewed several times (Whitten's paper[48] is a succinct and accessible recent statement) and will not be dealt with at any length here. Suffice it to say that in many cases testing has been harmful, uninformative, coercive, misleading and chaotic. There are, of course, exceptions, and well-organized programs are becoming more common as a result of recent publicity about the badly organized ones. But sickle cell screening is, by all accounts, a disastrous chapter in genetic screening's brief history, perhaps most of all because, like that for PKU, it has been written into law in several of our states.

The Laws

About a dozen states have passed sickle cell laws; several of them are either outright or ambiguously compulsory, though only two (those in Kentucky and Indiana) impose a penalty for noncompliance. Extensive discussion of their deficiencies is available elsewhere.[49,50] One of the most important things to note about these bills, however, is that they represent the initial venture into legislating heterozygote screening, and are thus viewed by some as an ominous sign that the government is attempting to set up criteria for childbearing. The fact that most legislators, including the bills' black sponsors, thought they were going after the disease rather than the carrier is irrelevant in this context: a vocal few persist in viewing any state involvement in minority reproduction as genocidal. Furthermore, since the options presented to sickle cell heterozygotes are generally directed toward preventing conception of any kind rather than preventing the birth of an affected child, it is not hard to understand why blacks – who, after all, *have* been the target of eugenic sterilization programs in this country – should be sensitive to such nuances. The charge of genocide has never been leveled against Tay-Sachs programs, despite the Jews' recent and all too memorable historical experience. That is almost certainly because they are voluntary and community-based rather than imposed, and because they can be presented as assuring the birth of only healthy children, which gives the impression of strengthening the community rather than decimating it. And usually no legislation is involved; it is a private, rather than a government, program.

Opponents of the laws have sometimes argued that they are unconstitutional, but there is a parade of previous compulsory public health measures that can be cited as precedent. In fact, genetic screening must have appeared similar to existing public health practices to many legislatures, because the laws are frequently amendments to existing statutes. Thus, for sickle cell disease, the regulations in nine states and the District of Columbia were added to extant requirements, such as preschool medical examinations and vaccinations and premarital venereal disease tests. (See the paper by Green and Capron in this series for a full treatment of the legal standing of compulsory screening laws.)

Most of the previously existing laws, of course, had been imposed to control that might be termed *horizontal* transmission of infectious disease, for instance, the requirement for smallpox vaccinations. The sickle cell laws seemed to represent a new attempt to control *vertical* transmission of genetic disease, but premarital sickle cell testing has a striking parallel in premarital blood testing for venereal disease, which has been required in some states since 1913.[51] Although venereal disease testing is chiefly justified on grounds that it prevents spread of disease from one sexual partner to another, the Supreme Court of Wisconsin recognized as early as 1914 that prevention of disease in children born of the relationship was an important reason for the test.* Compulsory preschool medical exams and immunizations are, of course, common, and were long ago held to be constitutional.[52] But preschool screening also has a kind of reverse precedent in rubella immunization, which is required in 22 states before school entry. Epidemiology is really quite emphatic in declaring that these laws are not as concerned with preventing the disease in those children immunized as they are with preventing infection of any of their mothers who might be pregnant. The target, as Hinman and Redmond[53] have recently pointed out, "is not the individual child but the fetus of a susceptible woman in the first two trimesters of gestation." This, too, might be called an effort to prevent vertical disease transmission. (It should be noted that there is currently a certain amount of medical disenchantment with the "herd immunity" principle marshaled to justify the procedure. Repeal of the compulsory rubella immunization laws has recently been advocated, on grounds that they have not really prevented spread of the disease to pregnant women.[54])

Those who fear state intervention in reproductive decisions can cite precedent too: 12 states prohibit marriage for the retarded,[55] and more than half the states have rarely enforced compulsory eugenic sterilization laws, dating back decades, still on their books.[56]

But as Grad[52] recently pointed out, "The power to order an individual to undergo a medical procedure – such as immunization – not, primarily, for his own health, but for the protection of the health and welfare of others, is a potentially far-reaching one." Furthermore, there are now so many kinds of compulsory health measures that we no longer even think of them as compulsory; in some cases, we even seek them out.

It seems quite clear that the intent of the present laws is not nearly as Machiavellian as some critics have said; they represent benign, if misguided, attempts to deal with health problems that seemed to their sponsors to be urgent. However, their consequences, particularly those of

---

*"The power of the state to control and regulate by reasonable laws the marriage relation, and to prevent the contracting of marriage by persons afflicted with loathsome or hereditary diseases, which are liable either to be transmitted to the spouse or inherited by the offspring, or both, must on principle be regarded as undeniable." (*Peterson vs. Widule,* 157 Wis. 641, 147 N.W. 966, 1914, quoted by Tobey, 1947.)

the sickle cell laws, have led to some agitation for repeal, or at least amendment. (In this context, it is perhaps worth noting that many of the laws on the books are not being enforced. In some cases this is because they were never funded. In others, public outcry restrained enforcement.) At least one state, Maryland, has repealed its original sickle cell law and tried a different tack. Maryland's approach is to date unique.

In the spring of 1972, the Maryland state senate passed into law a sickle cell bill that was a little more sensible than most. It did not demand compulsory testing. Instead it specified that information about the disease and the availability of tests and counseling be provided to applicants for a marriage license, and directed that all participation be voluntary. It made clear distinctions between the sickle cell trait and the disease. It directed that free testing be available in each health district and provided strong protection for record confidentiality. It even set up an advisory committee of unpaid "consumers of health services" to help the health department formulate its sickle cell information services.

In fact, the only really peculiar feature of this bill was an amendment stating, "If a blood test is administered to a pregnant female upon entering a hospital for delivery, the blood test shall include a test for sickle cell anemia" (Sect. 33A, Art. 43, Chap. 490, Maryland Statues of 1972). The fuzzy rationale for that addition was presumably the fact that many women with the disease are, not surprisingly, at greater risk in childbirth than the women without it.[57] It would, however, be very rare indeed for a woman with sickle cell anemia to remain undiagnosed for so long. A detailed examination of most of the state laws makes it clear, however, that they were drafted to scoop up people at various points of existing contact with state health systems, with little regard for what time of life might be medically sensible. It is obviously a good deal easier (and cheaper) to tack one more test onto an extant procedure, a marriage license blood test for instance, than to formulate and put into practice an entirely new set of machinery, such as widespread genetic education and testing in junior high school, an alternative proposed by some advocates of screening.[49]

Maryland's sickle cell bill was special because the senator who sponsored the original bill, Julian Lapides, had the assistance of the Eagleton Institute of Politics at Rutgers, which gives state legislators help in researching and drafting legislation. Following public criticism of the sickle cell laws, a new, more general law was drawn up, also with the Eagleton Institute's help. The result was a lengthy, careful bill (Chap. 695, Maryland Statutes of 1973) that attempts to meet all the criticisms leveled at other genetic screening bills. Essentially, it establishes a 16-member commission on hereditary disorders. The commission, composed of nonmedical appointees, doctors and members of the state health department, has a number of powers. For instance, it can establish regulations for detection and management of hereditary disorders, it can control information about them and it can even investigate charges of unjustified discrimination as a result of them. There are also strong provisions for protection of confidentiality of records and for availability of counseling services. A lengthy preamble makes a number of points to justify the commission; among them is the notion that we are all carriers, and that stigmatization of such a carrier is unjustified. The preamble also states unequivocally that "each person in the state of Maryland is entitled to the highest level of health care attainable, and to protection from inadequate health services not in the person's best interest." Interestingly, however, another declaration – "that the extremely personal decision to bear children, should remain the free choice and responsibility of the individual, and that such free choice and responsibility should not be restricted by the state" – was stricken from the final version of the bill. That paragraph was rejected partially at the behest of foes of legalized abortion, but it is also plausible to speculate that the legislators could foresee a time when they might find it desirable to restrict childbearing.

The new bill also provided for the repeal of both of the previous Maryland genetic screening bills, those dealing with sickle cell and PKU. The sickle cell repeal cleared easily. The effort to repeal the PKU bill, however, was beaten; thus Maryland still requires its newborns to be tested for PKU.

Until the commission has been in operation for a while, there is no way to tell whether it will simply add another layer of bureaucracy to the existing picture. The commission approach is likely to be used elsewhere, since a bill almost identical to the one in Maryland (but retaining the right-to-bear-children clause) was presented to a conference sponsored by the Council of State Governments early in the summer of 1973. There it was adopted as model legislation on genetic matters, and will be available to other state legislatures as a guideline.

The nub of this proposal, the advisory commission, was contained in the previous Maryland sickle cell bill, which also established such a group. But the idea of an advisory commission originated in the first modern law (Chap. 572, Minnesota Session Laws, 1959) dealing specifically with public health aspects of genetic disease (excluding the eugenic sterilization laws passed early in this century, which seem to be rather a different case).

The preamble of the Minnesota law indicates that it was, at least in part, a response to a common concern in that heyday of fallout shelters – worry over radiation damage. It authorized the Minnesota state health department to collect data, disseminate information and provide counseling services, and also set up a nine-member advisory committee on problems of human genetics, to assist the health department in its decisions about the kind of work to be done.

One advantage to the advisory commission approach may turn out, oddly enough, to be the very ponderousness of such bureaucratic machinery. All previous legislation had been a hasty, scattershot, impulsive response to what seemed to its sponsors like an urgent problem. The commission pathway is likely to be a good deal more deliberate. Such slow, thoughtful consideration before instituting a program might give us a chance to learn from past mistakes and keep us from making others in the future. On the other hand, despite its commission, Minnesota has a PKU law. It does not have a sickle cell law, but that is probably largely due to its numerically small black population. Kittrie[1] observes:

> If legislatures remain cautious, the authority for social experiments in human modification will rest with the administrative level, even though it is highly undesirable for drastic state power over procreation or other human modification to be invoked by experts and administrators without prior legislative deliberation and enactment.

On the other hand, while it is true, historically, that legislative bodies have occasionally saved us from our excesses, the legislative record in genetic matters is something less than encouraging. Kittrie believes these matters will – and in fact should – be settled in court:

> The future battles for the modification of man will therefore undoubtedly be fought in the judicial arena. . . .
>
> If the individual's right to be left alone is to be protected, the searchlight of public scrutiny must be focused upon this long-ignored power to modify man. The traditional Anglo-American tools of judicial process and review provide some of the most effective means for scrutiny known in any social system.

Genetic screening has not yet come that far.

It can certainly be argued that genetic screening laws could have valid functions. They could, for instance, enforce minimum screening standards, or assure that benefits are available to everyone. Since it appears likely that the laws will proliferate, it should be worthwhile to examine in detail what some of those functions could be.

In fact, genetic screening legislation provides an extraordinary opportunity to begin dealing with some serious but neglected issues in public health law in general. The most important one is protection of confidentiality, which has not to date been properly safeguarded in public health situations.[58] This concern grows more urgent with the proliferation of data banks. Record linkage has been held to be a key to meeting the challenge of genetic disease and congenital malformations, and has been experimented with in Canada and elsewhere.[59] One recent example is the Oxford (England) record linkage study,[60] which demonstrated an association between maternal epilepsy and congenital malformations. Its research and treatment benefits appear to be undeniable. But building in safeguards so that families are protected from possible harrassment should be among the chief considerations in drawing up such plans. Protection of computerized records does seem to be technically possible.[61] Genetic screening legislation might be one important way of helping assure that protection.

Some extant legislation has already dealt with this problem. The new Maryland law, for instance, requires that results be considered part of the confidential medical record (which place it in the protected doctor-patient category, rather than the relatively accessible public health category), and further specifies that the information be stored in code. The New York law (Public Health Law, Art. 27-C) establishing that state's much-admired Birth Defects Institute (which collects information on all types of congenital malformations, environmental and inherited), also contains a strong statement on protection of records: "Such reports and information shall be kept confidential and shall not be admissible as evidence in an action or proceeding in any court or before any other tribunal, board, agency or person." But most of the laws simply ignore the issue.

The screening laws could also set up machinery for careful, realistic public education about genetic disease. Sorenson[62] has pointed out that people get their information about genetic disease from outside their usual sources of medical information, which are the media and their doctors. Most genetic information results from contact with affected family members or friends. Further, genetic counseling and screening have historically been the privilege of the upper and middle classes.[62] Well-drawn laws could increase public knowledge (and demand) and thus could initiate more equitable distribution of these services. In addition, better education might help encourage voluntary participation in screening programs, thus lessening the justification for compulsory laws. There are some data (from nongenetic screening programs) supporting the argument that a properly designed program increases public knowledge about health and decreases anxiety about it.[63]

At some point, the laws are probably going to have to tackle the thorny and politically unattractive matter of race and ethnic classification, along with protection of minority rights. As tests proliferate, it will soon be quite clear that it is spendthrift to test people for conditions they almost certainly do not have. On the matter of race, current legislation is sometimes devious to the point of being comic. New York State is probably the best example. Its preschool sickle cell screening law specified the testing of children "in a city school district contained within a city" (Chaps. 903 and 904, Art. 19); the premarital screening law directs that tests be administered to those who are "not of the Caucasian, Indian or Oriental race" (Chap. 994, Sect. 13 aa, Session Law 1972).

The laws should also provide machinery for setting up and enforcing medical standards for screening. But those standards must be flexible enough to allow for rapidly changing technology in this field, and should not be too specific about particular tests to use. In this area, the advisory committee approach is probably very sensible.

Some Other Effects

One of the most interesting outgrowths of genetic screening to date has been confirmation of our heterogeneity, in both health and disease. Newborn screening has revealed that PKU is not a single entity. An Ontario study,[27] for instance, found that a third of its cases were "atypical" PKU. Putting infants with mild hyperphenylalanemia on the special diet has resulted in death from phenylalanine deficiency. Even when it is not physically harmful, the diet is very disruptive to family life and should never be needlessly imposed.[64] Adult phenylketonurics with normal intelligence have also been found.[65] Mild sickle cell disease is fairly common,[66] and a kindred with apparent absence of hexosaminidase A in perfectly healthy adults has also been reported.[67] One lesson to be drawn from these data is cautionary. It militates against an assembly-line procedure for uniform treatment of conditions that turn out not to be uniform. The other side of the coin may be something of a comfort to champions of the individual in an age of conformity. We really are all unique: in our fingerprints, our biochemistry and even our disease.

There is another possible effect; it is moot, but there are some data to support it. Can the knowledge that one is a carrier of a serious disease be so personally disruptive that the harm outweighs any possible benefit? Such harm, if it exists, may not be completely a function of how well or poorly organized the screening is. Another paper in this series[68] points out that we don't yet know all the social and psychologic risks in screening, that parameter has remained largely uninvestigated.

One exception is a follow-up study by Stamatoyannopoulos[69] and his colleagues of a 3½-year screening program for sickle cell heterozygotes in the small Greek village of Orchomenos. This population is exceptionally sickle cell conscious because the carrier frequency is 23% and the newborn disease incidence about 1 in 100. Yet this carefully designed and executed program still resulted in four carrier-carrier marriages. The prescreening expected number was only 4.5. Furthermore, there was some social cost. Engagements were disrupted and prevented. People did feel stigmatized enough so that they lied about their status to prospective mates. It might be argued that these anxieties would be justified by reduction of the number of heterozygote marriages. Since that goal was not accomplished, the entire project appears discouraging, futile and possibly actively harmful.

It can certainly be argued that events in a small Greek village, where marriages are arranged in lengthy family negotiations, may have very little application here, any more than does Italian screening for thalassemia. But the story is arresting nonetheless, and certainly argues the need for such a long-term follow-up on U. S. programs. This kind of disruption of social life may be peculiar to a disease like sickle cell, where the options are so limited. Even Cohen,[63] who thinks anxiety generated by mass screening programs is justified if the programs result in treatment, concedes, "If we do not have such criteria, then we have no right to arouse anxiety in the community." The argument thus hinges on whether reduction of the number of carrier-carrier marriages constitutes treatment, and whether (in light of the Greek data) such treatment is a realistic goal. But there may be unexpected anxieties raised even when prenatal diagnosis is available.

The Future

It is already possible to discern a few trends in genetic screening and get an idea of what the future is likely to hold.

First, and most predictable, screening will be extended in a number of ways. More carrier tests and prenatal diagnoses will be developed. As this is being written, an improved heterozygote screening procedure for cystic fibrosis[70] is in the offing, and there is hope for prenatal diagnosis. This is the most common "white" recessive disease, and occurs in about 1 in 2,500 live births in that group. Areas of heavy Mediterranean population have begun to demand thalassemia screening; a pilot program, offered to members of two Greek Orthodox churches, has been conducted.[71] A bill providing for treatment of thalassemia, and another for hemophilia, has been considered in New Jersey. How long will legislators pay for treatment without requiring screening? As technics permit, testing for other, rarer conditions will also become available, and affected groups will clamor for them, particularly if they follow the Tay-Sachs model in providing a variety of alternatives.

Further, mass prenatal diagnosis will probably become part of genetic screening. A recent proposal by Stein, Susser and Guterman[72] predicts the virtual eradication of the Down syndrome (mongolism), the single most important cause of mental retardation, if amniocentesis is made a part of routine prenatal care. They propose a four-phase plan, beginning with all pregnant women over age 40, the most at-risk group. Harper[73] has pointed out that this is already routine at some centers. There are certainly many logistic and ethical problems with such a sweeping program, but it is bound to seem increasingly attractive both to nervous prospective parents and to legislators who must somehow keep finding money for state institutions for the retarded. Routine karyotyping for trisomy 21 would also reveal all the other chromosome aneuploidies. If the newest staining technics are used, the karyotypes will also begin to reveal those previously less obvious chromosome aberrations that are beginning to be catalogued and associated with various syndromes as a result of those new technics. Biochemical tests may also be run on those same cells. In Edwards'[74] opinion:

> Since amniotic cells cannot be obtained without risk a strong case can be made that they should be screened for any other abnormality which can be detected with precision. Tay-Sachs disease, although virtually restricted to Ashkenazi Jews, should certainly be included in New York, and any plan which left out the problems of sickle cell anemia and thalassemia, which, in some racial groups, are commoner than mongolism and even more distressing, would seem unsatisfactory.

Once again the programs will be aimed at prevention of the person rather than the disease, but it may be that such distinctions will not be apparent to most people. Or that families anxious to avoid abnormality will brush the distinctions aside. As abortion-on-demand becomes more acceptable, drawing up rules for medical abortions will begin to seem pointless.

Another extension of screening will come with the virtual disappearance of the single-gene programs commonly thought of as "genetic screening." Already the trend is apparent. The newborn screening program in Massachusetts has already been mentioned; New York and other states are following suit.

A recent New York City area pilot program combined screening for Tay-Sachs disease with that for hyperlipidemia (G. Sachs, personal communication, 1973). This search for elevated blood lipids and cholesterol represents an interesting departure: the condition is not especially more common among Jews than among other ethnic groups, but the screening is an attempt to alert and educate those people who may be particularly at risk for cardiovascular disease in later life, and the Tay-Sachs blood sample offers easy access to a relatively common presymptomatic state. A program of this kind opens up the vast area of euphenics, in which the genetically susceptible can take steps to alter their environment in an effort to prevent degenerative changes decades before they might normally occur. At the heart of this move is our changing definition of illness:

> Should diseases be likened to ivy growing on the oak tree or are they part of the oak tree itself? Should diseases be regarded as human analogues of defects in an internal-combustion engine or a Swiss watch, or should they be regarded as psychobiological expressions of man evolving within the constraints and potentials contributed from his aliquot of society's gene pool? Are diseases "things" that "happen" to people, or are they manifestations of constructive or destructive relations of individuals in their social and physical environment?[2]

This latter view of all disease as potential, and dependent for its development on a push from its surroundings, has been praised as the last great challenge left to medicine. Yet it is curiously similar to a world-view that Western medicine long ago dismissed as primitive, the view that disease is, at bottom, the expression of an individual's disharmony with nature.

Those examples are at least more or less genetic, but genetic screening is also being combined with testing for nongenetic conditions. There is at least one hospital-based sickle cell screening program in New York that has tested its blood samples for all kinds of anemia as well as abnormal hemoglobins (C. Sinnette, personal communication, 1973). This kind of program represents one way of gaining entry to some crushing (and much more common) health problems of the community, and is surely not unique. In fact, the possibility of bootlegging a more adequate general health program in the guise of a sickle cell program is certainly one reason why the programs have not been criticized even more strongly, or abandoned altogether. Some attention paid to black health – even if it has some disadvantages – is better than none at all.[43]

Programs like these are likely to blur the distinctions many people make between genetic and nongenetic disorders; genetic screening will simply become part of the mass screening picture. Indeed, it can be argued that screening for conditions like diabetes and hypertension, which has been going on for some time, is genetic screening too. But as long as genetic screening is regarded by many as somehow different and especially sensitive, it will remain controversial. The very sensitivity of the issues, however, and the caution with which it now appears such screening must be handled, can also provide a unique opportunity for an attack on some serious and so far unsolved problems in public health.

Conclusion

Is it possible to discern some common factors in these disparate approaches to genetic health? If there is some confluence of external conditions that has in the past led to the institution of genetic screening, can that pattern repeat itself in the future? This paper will conclude by arguing that there are such conditions, that they can be identified and that they are proliferating, but that their identification can be a tool for anticipating (and preventing) the possible harmful consequences of new screening programs.

The first such condition leading to the introduction of a new screening program is, of course, a relatively simple and cheap test that will detect a biochemical variant. In another paper in this series, Lappé and Roblin[75] demonstrate how rapidly the number of such procedures is increasing. These new procedures must be judged in light of an extensive modern literature[76,77] arguing that technology provides its own impetus, irrespective of and uncontrolled by human agency. Medicine in general and genetic screening in particular can provide excellent examples to bolster those arguments. The mere existence of a test somehow serves as its own justification. It is regrettably true that, just because we *can* do something, we very often proceed to do it, without thinking much about whether we *should*. Ellul[76] has observed:

> The rules obeyed by a technical organization are no longer rules of justice or injustice. They are "laws" in a purely technical sense . . . neither economic nor political evolution conditions technical progress. Its progress is likewise independent of the social situation . . . Technique elicits and conditions social, political and economic change.

According to Bennett, "Analysis of the problems of medical care must *precede* solution. It will not suffice to *adapt* the problems to an existing set of methods or technologies."[78] Such judgements seem exceptionally applicable to development of tests for genetic screening.

As a corollary, it is important to point out that the test in question need *not* be a very good test. The literature is dotted with arguments about the merits and demerits of screening procedures. The U. S. Public Health Service's Center for Disease Control, for instance, evaluated[79] a number of commercial solubility tests for hemoglobin S and found their accuracy quite variable and their labeling and insert information often incomplete and inaccurate. These preparations are among the most flagrant, but not the only, examples of inadequate genetic screening tests.[12,13] Thus, in addition to appearing to have life and momentum of its own, technology compounds its attendant disadvantages by being so often imperfect. At least some of the damage it does can be traced to its failures, rather than to its successes.

A second requirement for genetic screening is a disease, or some kind of collection of conditions that it is possible to think of as a disease. That is not quite so straightforward as it may first appear. Doctors know how heterogeneous the ailments they deal with really are, even when the variants are called by a single name. Genetic diseases are notoriously variable.[13,27] Some diseases do not even exist in our minds or our textbooks *as* diseases until after we can test for them. A recent example is adenosine deaminase deficiency, which is thought to be an inherited immune-deficiency disease now that the enzyme's absence can be detected. The first case reports[80] appeared late in 1972, after a test had been devised; but less than a year later there was talk of adding the test, by compulsory law, to the newborn screening program in New York State. It is critical to our thinking and planning (such as it is) to be able to deal with a named entity, and we can move very quickly once we have given the enemy its name.

Strickland[81] has documented as a political event the rise of the medical research establishment in this country, largely as a result of our support of attacks on "cancer" and "heart disease." Genetic screening is quite clearly an example of what has been called this "category" approach to disease. Ebert[82] and others have pointed out that even our supra-medical agency betrays this approach in its name: the National Institutes of Health. Such an approach, while it may have some impact on individual diseases, undoubtedly fragments our resources and works against rational overall planning. Researchers who need funding and lay persons who want to "do something" about the disease (not infrequently because they or their relatives have it) are intimately involved in constructing these categorizations. The process is circular and self-perpetuating: money is available for very specific purposes; so projects are designed for narrow goals in order to qualify for that money. Despite all our recent talk of reordering our priorities, money is not available for such reordering and planning; so it does not get done. Fields like genetic screening grow haphazardly as we set out in several directions at once.

The third factor critical to institution of screening is researchers (and research needs), for whom mass screening is a way of getting data (particularly on very rare conditions) that are simply unavailable otherwise. Furthermore, in the case of a disease like PKU, screening provides virtually the only testing ground for a new therapy or, as in Tay-Sachs, a new technic. On the other hand, it is also possible for health professionals to combine to resist introduction of a new procedure, as they did PKU screening in one area of Washington State. Usually, however, the better the local physician communication, the faster screening is adopted.[15]

Bessman and Swazey have pointed to the involvement of researchers, foundations and government officials in the genesis of PKU screening. The original Baltimore-Washington Tay-Sachs program was run by researchers at Johns Hopkins, the John F. Kennedy Institute Tay-Sachs Fund, the Aaron and Lillian Strauss Foundation and the Maryland State Department of Health and Mental Hygiene.[30] Even while denouncing the sickle cell laws, health professionals in that field have sometimes clung to them, because they mean money and attention devoted, at long last, to black health problems.[43] Screening unqestionably serves research interests. It has been said (H. L. Levy, personal communication, 1973), for instance, that we only know as much as we do about PKU because we screen for it. Research is a rational, legitimate and honest purpose of screening, but in that case, perhaps it is both dishonest and unwise to present screening as having service as its chief objective. Unwittingly or not, genetic screening has been historically portrayed as therapeutic (perhaps because the formal validation procedures have always insisted that treatment be a goal of screening). However, the therapies have often been inadequate, or even nonexistent, and this is surely at the heart of public disappointment.

The last factor contributing to screening is a group of laymen with some interest and involvement.[82] Frequently, this has meant relatives of people with the disease in question, as in PKU, where relatives provided part of the political pressure that led to the laws.[12] Sometimes, as in Tay-Sachs, it has meant groups with strong ties to the community; once alerted they become eager proselytizers for screening.[30] In sickle cell it has been black legislators, who viewed the laws they sponsored not as compelling little children to suffer feelings of inadequacy and confusion, but as *compelling the state* to make a start toward solving some long-neglected health problems in the black community.[49] Sometimes the center of this interest has been a formal organization, which acts as a focus of concern (and money), as a spokesman and as a pressure group. The organization, however, is generally formed as a response to demand rather than prior to it. It can also contribute to the harm that is done. Sickle Cell Anemia Research & Education, Inc., for instance, emphasizes its acronym in its publicity materials. It is hard to see how the word SCARE can reassure an anxious screenee. This kind of lay involvement has frequently been overlooked as an important factor in the institution of new medical procedures. It may turn out to be particularly crucial for genetic medicine, which is by definition ethnic and therefore has a number of ready-made constituencies, particularly in this country.

Social and technologic forces can achieve a fearsome synergy, as the continuing history of genetic screening – and perhaps all of modern medicine[83] – demonstrates. Perhaps this is particularly true because the motives behind it are demonstrably benign. What Bessman and Swazey said about PKU applies equally to other genetic screening: it is not a question of bad faith; those who have pushed for screening "simply identified their own interest with the public interest."[12] Like so many other treatments with unanticipated side-effects, like so many other ventures of the therapeutic state, genetic screening has always seemed a good idea at the time.

Acknowledgment

The author is grateful for suggestions from Marc Lappé, Peter Steinfels, Richard Roblin and, especially, James M. Gustafson.

References

1. Kittrie, N. N.: *The Right to be Different.* Baltimore and London:The Johns Hopkins Press, 1971.
2. White, K. L.: Life and death and medicine. *Sci. Amer., 229*:23, 1973.
3. Wilson, J. M. G. and Jungner, G.: *Principles and Practice of Screening for Disease.* Geneva:World Health Organization, 1968.
4. Wain, H.: *A History of Preventive Medicine.* Springfield:Charles C Thomas, 1970.
5. Pole, J. D.: The cost-effectiveness of screening. *Proc. Roy. Soc. Med., 64*:1256, 1971.
6. Glazier, W. H.: The task of medicine. *Sci. Amer., 228*:13, 1973.
7. Black, M. M. and Riley, C.: Moral issues and priorities in biomedical engineering. *Sci. Med. Man., 1*:67, 1973.

8. Cochrane, A. L. and Holland, W. W.: Validation of screening procedures. *Brit. Med. Bull., 27*:3, 1971.
9. Powles, J.: On the limitations of modern medicine. *Sci. Med. Man., 1*:1, 1973.
10. McKeown, T.: Validation of screening procedures. In *Screening in Medical Care.* London:Oxford University Press, 1968.
11. Nitowsky, H. M.: Prescriptive screening for inborn errors of metabolism: A critique. *Amer. J. Ment. Defic., 77*:538, 1973.
12. Bessman, S. P. and Swazey, J. P.: PKU: A study of biomedical legislation. In Mendelsohn, E., Swazey, J. P., and Taviss, I. (eds.): *Human Aspects of Biomedical Innovation.* Cambridge:Harvard University Press, 1971.
13. Cunningham, G. C.: Phenylketonuria testing – Its role in pediatrics and public health. *CRC Crit. Rev. Clin. Lab. Sci., 2*:45, 1971.
14. Paulissen, J. P. and Zeldes, M.: PKU program in Illinois: A 10-year study, *Illinois Med. J., 140*:583, 1971.
15. Holm, V. A., Deering, W. M. and Penn, R. L.: Some factors influencing the development of a voluntary PKU screening program: Possible implication for other screening procedures for newborns. *JAMA, 212*:1835, 1970.
16. *Screening for Inborn Errors of Metabolism.* Technical Reprint Series, No. 401, World Health Organization, 1968.
17. Scriver, C. R.: Screening for inherited traits: Perspectives. In Harris, M. (ed.): *Early Diagnosis of Human Genetic Defects: Fogarty International Center Proceedings No. 6,* Department of Health, Education and Welfare, 1970.
18. Shih, V. E. and Levy, H. L.: Cost-benefit of neonate screening. *New Eng. J. Med., 285*:240, 1971.
19. Levy, H. L.: Newborn screening for metabolic disorders. *New Eng. J. Med., 288*:1299, 1973.
20. Shih, V. E., Levy, H. L., Karolkewicz, V. et al: Galactosemia screening of newborns in Massachusetts. *New Eng. J. Med., 284*:753, 1971.
21. Levy, H. L. and Shih, V. E.: Screening for galactosemia. *New Eng. J. Med., 287*:723, 1972.
22. Ellis, G., Wilcock, A. R. and Goldberg, D. M.: Experience of routine live birth screening for galactosemia in a British hospital with emphasis on heterozygote detection. *Arch. Dis. Child., 47*:34, 1972.
23. Bradley, G. M.: Urinary screening tests in the infant and young child. *Med. Clin. N. Amer., 55*:1457, 1971.
24. Garrick, M. D., Dembure, P. and Guthrie, R.: Sickle cell anemia and other hemoglobinopathies, procedures and strategy for screening employing spots of blood on filter paper as specimens. *New Eng. J. Med., 288*:1265, 1973.
25. Raine, D. N., Cooke, J. R., Andrews, W. A. and Mahon, D. F.: Screening for inherited metabolic disease by plasma chromotography (Scriver) in a large city *Brit. Med. J., 3*:7, 1972.
26. Clow, C. L., Fraser, F. C., Laberge, C. and Scriver, C. R.: On the application of knowledge to the patient with genetic disease. *Prog. Med. Genet., 9*:159, 1973.
27. Advisory Committee on Inborn Errors of Metabolism to the Ministry of Health: PKU screening – Is it worth it? *Can. Med. Ass. J., 108*:328, 1973.
28. Hook, E. B.: Behavioral implications of the human XYY genotype. *Science, 179*:139, 1973.

29. Kass, L. R.: Implication of prenatal diagnosis for the human right to life. In Hilton, B., Callahan, D., Harris, M. et al (eds.): *Ethical Issues in Human Genetics.* New York and London:Plenum Press, 1973.
30. Kaback, M. M. and Zeiger, R. S.: The John F. Kennedy Institute Tay-Sachs Program: Practical and ethical issues in an adult genetic screening program. In Hilton, B., Callahan, D., Harris, M. et al (eds.): *Ethical Issues in Human Genetics.* New York and London:Plenum Press, 1973.
31. Motulsky, A. G.: Frequency of sickling disorder in U. S. blacks. *New Eng. J. Med., 288*:31, 1973.
32. Scott, R. R.: Health care priority and sickle cell anemia. *JAMA, 214*:731, 1970.
33. Gelpi, A. P. and Perrine, R. P.: Sickle cell disease and trait in white populations. *JAMA, 224*:605, 1973.
34. McGrew, C. J.: Sickle cell trait in the white population. *JAMA, 224*:1762, 1973.
35. Pearson, H. A. and O'Brien, R. T.: Sickle cell testing programs. *J. Pediat., 81*:1201, 1972.
36. Valenti, C.: Antenatal detection of hemoglobinopathies. *Amer. J. Obstet. Gynec., 115*:851, 1973.
37. Ramsey, P.: Screening: An ethicist's view. In Hilton, B., Callahan, D., Harris, M. et al (eds.): *Ethical Issues in Human Genetics.* New York and London:Plenum Press, 1973.
38. *Human Genetics and Public Health,* Technical Reprint Series, #282, World Health Organization, 1964.
39. Jones, S. R., Binder, R. A. and Donowho, E. M., Jr.: Sudden death in sickle cell trait. *New Eng. J. Med., 282*:323, 1970.
40. Mosher, M. B.: Sickle cell trait. *New Eng. J. Med., 282*:1157, 1970.
41. *The S-Hemoglobinopathies: An Evaluation of their Status in Armed Forces.* National Academy of Sciences-National Research Council, 1973.
42. Murphy, J. R.: Sickle cell hemoglobin (hemoglobin AS) in black football players. *JAMA, 225*:981, 1973.
43. Culliton, B. J.: Sickle cell anemia: National program raises problems as well as hopes. *Science, 178*:283, 1972.
44. Disease Detection Information Bureau: *The Role of Community Organizations in Disease Screening Programs.* Proceedings of a conference, New York City, June 11-12, 1971.
45. Feldman, J. J.: *The Dissemination of Health Information.* Chicago:Aldine Publishing Company, 1966.
46. Kaback, M. M., Becker, M. H. and Ruth, M. V.: Sociological studies in human genetics: I. Compliance factors in a voluntary heterozygote screening program. (This volume.)
47. Bowman, J. E.: Mass screening programs for sickle hemoglobin: A sickle cell crisis. *JAMA, 222*:1650, 1972.
48. Whitten, C. F.: Sickle cell programming – An imperiled promise. *New Eng. J. Med., 288*:318, 1973.
49. Powledge, T.: The new ghetto hustle. *Saturday Review of the Sciences*, Jan. 27, 1973.
50. Reilly, P.: Sickle cell anemia legislation. *J. Legal Med., 1*:4:39; 1:5:36, 1973.
51. Tobey, J. A.: *Public Health Law.* New York:The Commonwealth Fund, 1947.

52. Grad, F. P.: *Public Health Law Manual.* The American Public Health Association, 1970.
53. Hinman, A. R. and Redmond, S.: Efficacy of rubella immunizations. *New Eng. J. Med., 288*:1357, 1973.
54. Weinstein, L. and Chang, T. W.: Rubella immunization. *New Eng. J. Med., 288*:100, 1973.
55. Krishef, C. H.: State laws on marriage and sterilization of the mentally retarded. *Ment. Retard., 10*:36, 1972.
56. Holder, A. R.: Compulsory sterilization. *JAMA, 221*:229, 1972.
57. Fort, A. T.: Counseling patients with sickle cell disease about reproduction: Pregnancy outcome does not justify the maternal risk! *Amer. J. Obstet. Gynec., 111*:324, 1971.
58. Schwitzgebel, R. K.: Confidentiality of research information in public health studies. *Harvard Legal Comment., 6*:187, 1969.
59. Newcombe, H. B.: Record linkage – Its role in congenital defect research. In Porter, I. and Skalko, R. G. (eds.): *Congenital Defects,* Proceedings of the Birth Defects Institute, October 1972, Albany, N. Y. New York:Academic Press, 1974.
60. Fedrick, J.: Epilepsy and pregnancy: A report from the Oxford record linkage study. *Brit. Med. J., 2*:442, 1973.
61. Feistel, H.: Cryptography and computer privacy. *Sci. Amer., 228*:15, 1973.
62. Sorenson, J. R.: *Social Aspects of Applied Human Genetics.* New York:Russell Sage Foundation, 1971.
63. Cohen, S. I.: The psychiatric effects of mass screening. *Public Health, 86*:125, 1972.
64. Buist, N. R. and Jhaveri, B. M.: A guide to screening newborn infants for inborn errors of metabolism. *J. Pediat., 82*:511, 1973.
65. Perry, T. L., Hansen, S., Tischler, B. et al: Unrecognized adult phenylketonuria: Implications for obstetrics and psychiatry. *New Eng. J. Med., 289*:395, 1973.
66. Steinberg, M. H., Dreiling, B. J., Morrison, F. S. and Necheles, T. F.: Mild sickle cell disease: Clinical and laboratory studies. *JAMA, 224*:317, 1973.
67. Navon, R., Padeh, B. and Adam, A.: Apparent deficiency of hexosaminidose A in healthy members of a family with Tay-Sachs disease. *Amer. J. Hum. Genet., 25*:287, 1973.
68. Fletcher, J., Roblin, R. D. and Powledge, T. M.: Informed consent in genetic screening programs. (This volume.)
69. Stamatoyannopoulos, G.: Problems of screening and counseling in the hemoglobinopathies. Read at the Fourth International Conference on Birth Defects, Vienna, Austria, Sept. 2-8, 1973.
70. Bearn, A. G.: Cell culture in inherited disease – With some notes on genetic heterogeneity. *New Eng. J. Med., 286*:764, 1972.
71. Pearson, H. A., O'Brien, R. T. and McIntosh, S.: Screening for thalassemia trait by electronic measurement of mean corpuscular volume. *New Eng. J. Med., 288*:351, 1973.
72. Stein, Z., Susser, M. and Guterman, A. V.: Screening programme for prevention of Down's syndrome. *Lancet, 1*:305, 1973.
73. Harper, P. S.: The prenatal diagnosis of metabolic disorders. *J. Roy. Coll. Physicians Lond., 7*:251, 1973.

74. Edwards, J. H.: Screening for chromosome abnormalities. *Lancet, 1*:542, 1973.
75. Lappé, M. and Roblin, R.: Newborn genetic screening as a concept in health care delivery: A critique. (This volume.)
76. Ellul, J.: *The Technological Society.* New York: Alfred A. Knopf, 1964.
77. Callahan, D.: *The Tyranny of Survival.* New York: MacMillan Publishing Co., Inc., 1973.
78. Bennett, I. L.: The future of preventive medicine. *Arch. Environ. Health, 19*:419, 1969.
79. Schmidt, R. M. and Wilson, S. M.: Standardization in detection of abnormal hemoglobins. *JAMA, 225*:1225, 1973.
80. Giblett, E. R., Anderson, J. E., Cohen, F. et al: Adenosine-deaminase deficiency in two patients with severely impaired cellular immunity. *Lancet, 2*:1067, 1972.
81. Strickland, S. P.: *Politics, Science and Dread Disease.* Cambridge: Harvard U. Press, 1972.
82. Ebert, R. H.: Biomedical research policy – A re-evaluation. *New Eng. J. Med., 289*:348, 1973.
83. White, K. L., Murnaghan, J. H. and Gaus, C. R.: Technology and health care. *New Eng. J. Med., 287*:1223, 1972.

Issues of Law and Public Policy in Genetic Screening

Harold P. Green, J.D. and Alexander M. Capron, LL.B.

The growing ability of medical science to diagnose asymptomatic inherited disorders plainly has great implications for health care and decisions about reproduction. As diagnostic capabilities are perfected and semiautomated, so that they are reliable, fast and economical, physicians, private organizations and governmental agencies will become interested in the mass application of these technics – indeed, large-scale screening programs have already been launched in some places for genetic diseases. In addition to the implications for medicine and reproduction, mass screening programs raise a host of important issues for law and public policy. In analyzing those issues, it is useful to begin by distinguishing between those screening programs which are voluntary and those which are mandatory.

Voluntary Screening Programs

In considering screening programs to which individuals submit voluntarily, a distinction may be drawn between programs conducted by private and public agencies. The former may be freely conducted unless they in some way violate a statutory prohibition or limitation, such as the restrictions placed on the practice of medicine. In contrast, the latter programs involve an expenditure of public funds and may generally be undertaken only if such use of public funds has been affirmatively authorized, either explicitly or implicitly, by statute; they must also be conducted subject to relevant statutory and constitutional limitations.

Harold P. Green, J.D., *Professor of Law and Director of the Law, Science and Technology Program, The National Law Center, George Washington University, Washington, D. C. and* Alexander M. Capron, LL.B., *Assistant Professor of Law, University of Pennsylvania, Philadelphia.*

Where a public agency makes funds available to a private agency, its screening program would probably be deemed, for at least some purposes, a program conducted by a public agency.

Screening by Private Agencies

No state has enacted legislation which specifically restricts or regulates private genetic screening programs. Such restrictions or regulations are likely to arise only if a legislature perceives abuse. For example, statutory controls might be imposed if it appears that the process of voluntary screening is injurious to the health of the screenee or the fetus.[1] Beyond such specific enactments, genetic screening is subject to each state's statutory limitations on the practice of medicine solely by licensed physicians and those under their supervision, to the extent that the genetic screening involves physical interventions necessary for diagnosis.[2]

Legal problems in connection with voluntary genetic screening programs are likely to arise primarily in connection with the use of information obtained as a result of the screening of the individual. Two distinct kinds of cases can be visualized: those arising out of the failure of the screening agency to disclose information to the person screened,[3] and those arising out of the disclosure of information to persons other than the person screened.[4]

There is no legal authority directly on point for either of these types of problems in the context of genetic screening. Beyond the general principles of contract law, the most closely analogous precedents with respect to disclosure of information produced in screening programs are to be found in the decisions relating to the physician-patient relationship, and it is likely that these precedents would be drawn upon by the courts in considering cases which arose from genetic screening programs. These precedents may not supply a complete answer, however. Liability in genetic screening programs may arise from acts which occur outside the one-to-one relationship of physician and patient; indeed, even though genetic screening programs will probably be conducted under the supervision of physicians, the screenee may never have personal contact with a physician. In such a case, the question would be presented whether a lay screener has a greater or a lesser duty than a physician to disclose the diagnosis to the screenee and not to disclose it to other persons. Therefore, the courts would probably also turn to cases which resulted from other kinds of screening programs in which the duties of persons besides physicians were discussed.

The Screenee's Right to Receive the Diagnosis

To decide whether a person who voluntarily submits to genetic screening by a private agency has a right to a factual statement of screening results, one must consider a number of factors. The first is the expectation of the parties – specifically, whether the individual screened could reasonably have believed that he would be given the results. In most instances the screening program will make an explicit representation concerning the means which will be used to notify the screenees of the screening diagnosis, and in other cases the expectation that results will be communicated to the screenee will be implicit since the obtaining of a diagnosis is the motivating purpose behind the screenee's participation. Therefore, if an explicit or implicit promise is made to the person screened that he will have the benefit of knowing the result, it would appear that he has a legal right to be informed of the result. On the other hand, if the individual were solicited to cooperate in a research project designed solely to gather statistical data, without any promise that he would benefit from the results, there would appear to be no obligation to give him the information. In sum, since the relationship between screener and screenee is in the nature of a contract, the screener's breach of his promise to disclose the results of the screening to the screenee would make the screener liable for the foreseeable injuries to the screenee and his or her offspring[5]; even when the "contract" is informal, it would fall within the principle that if the promisor should reasonably expect that the promisee will rely on the promise, the promisor will be liable to the promisee if he suffers injury because of his reliance.[6]

A second factor is the extent to which the law governing physicians would be applicable. When the agency conducting the screening has not explicitly promised to disclose the results to the screenee, the duty it owes the person screened may be defined by analogy to a physician's duty to disclose a diagnosis to his patient, if the screening is considered a medical procedure or if it is conducted in a manner which could reasonably give the screenee the impression that it will be governed by the standards of conduct which usually obtain in physician-patient relations. The cases establish the general principle that the diagnosis should always be disclosed to the patient, subject to certain exceptions. This rule favoring disclosure is based on the proposition that the physician's superior knowledge and skill is the foundation of the patient's trust and confidence in him, and that the relationship created thereby is a fiduciary one, placing on the physician the burden and duty of "full and complete" disclosure of all facts which materially affect the patient's interest.[7] The cases that establish this requirement generally concern the duty of the physician to ensure that a patient's "informed consent" to proposed treatment is given with full understanding of the risks and alternatives.[8] The reasoning behind the cases – that the patient is entitled to information about his own condition so as to be able to make knowledgeable choices – seems equally applicable to a situation involving the results of screening, which may have a major impact on many decisions made by the person screened. Indeed, in one of these recent "informed consent" cases, the court observed in dictum that "due care may require a physician perceiving symptoms of bodily abnormality to alert the patient to the condition."[9]

The exception to the rule of full disclosure is similarly based on the patient's trust in the physician and on the physician's expertise. Assuming an ongoing physician-patient relationship, a "therapeutic privilege" permits the physician to withhold certain information if in his judgment disclosure would be antitherapeutic.[10] The appropriateness of invoking the privilege was measured in each instance by the prevailing standards of medical treatment in the community. Lately, however, several leading courts have held that the patient has made out liability when he proves that a reasonable person would want the information that the physician withheld; he need not prove that the physician deviated from any standard of medical practice.[11] The requirement of full disclosure to allow the patient the opportunity to make an informed decision is set by law, except where an emergency exists or where the patient is incompetent. Moreover, the burden of proof is shifted to the physician to prove that the information withheld would, if disclosed, have rendered the patient unable "to dispassionately weigh the risks of refusing to undergo the recommended treatment."[12] Thus, while the precise issue has yet to be decided by the courts, it would appear that the "therapeutic privilege" to withhold a diagnosis is limited to those situations in which the physician is also recommending a treatment which he believes is very important for the patient's health. In a purely diagnostic setting, such as that of genetic screening, the privilege to withhold a diagnosis would thus not exist, at least not as a result of the law on physicians' rights and duties toward their patients. The fact that, given the current state of science, there may be no possibility for medical treatment following a positive diagnosis of a particular genetic disorder or carrier status has no bearing on the physician's duty to disclose the information to the screenee. So long as the facts indicate that the person screened expects to be informed and may rely on this expectation, the screening agency has a duty to disclose. In other words, the principles derived from the law on the physician-patient relationship lead to the same conclusion as those of the general law of contracts.

Where a screening program is conducted not by physicians but entirely by laymen, the duty to disclose a positive result would likely be held to arise also from the same source as in the context of the physician-patient relationship – reasonable expectations and reliance on the part of the individual screened. The lay screener's obligations are not determined by the physician-screener's, since both the duty of the latter to make full disclosure and his qualified right to withhold information are based on his medical role and expertise and on the trust the patient places in him as a physician. Thus, in such circumstances, reference has to be to the implicit or explicit terms of the agreement between screener and screenee. Insofar as the only purpose of testing is the ascertainment of information on which the screenee may then rely in making decisions about medical treatment or about whether to have children, it seems probable that if a screenee suffers damages because the screener failed to inform him of a positive result, the screener will be held liable. Situations could arise in which the screener would believe he had good reasons not to disclose, but he would bear a very heavy burden of justifying his action if challenged.

A further area where the problem of disclosure may possibly arise is genetic testing carried out during, for instance, the course of a hospital stay or as one of a number of tests in a clinic or doctor's office. If such testing is done without the patient's knowledge of either its nature or the result, the question of the screener's liability for nondisclosure would also most likely be decided in favor of the screenee if he is able to show that injury resulted from his reasonable reliance on those responsible for his physical and medical care to inform him completely about any matters concerning his health. Thus, both physicians[13] and employers who had their employees examined medically[14] have been held liable for failure to disclose information, such as a chest x ray being positive for tuberculosis. As in the case of a physician, although a private agency may have no duty to screen, once it undertakes the test and knows the results it will be liable for failing to disclose them since "[b]y remaining silent," it permits the screenee "to rely upon a tacit assurance of safety despite its knowledge of the existence of danger."[15]

In sum, where the person screened has a justifiable expectation that he will be informed of any positive results, then there is a duty on the screener (ie physician, layman or private agency) to disclose the information. A soundly formulated genetic screening program should therefore include a written statement to be given to all potential screenees describing, among other things, the purposes of the screening and the screening agency's policy with respect to disclosure of the results to the person screened. Such a statement would define the rights of the person screened and the duties of the screening agency, thereby minimizing or perhaps obviating the need to resolve a dispute according to uncertain common law precedents.

Disclosure to Third Persons of Screening Results

A second problem concerns the unauthorized disclosure of the results of genetic screening to third persons. Again, when screening is conducted by laymen the analogy to the doctor-patient relationship will be instructive although not necessarily controlling.

For screening performed by physicians, the starting point is the Hippocratic Oath which prohibits a physician from revealing matters that he learns about his patients "which ought not to be spoken of abroad." The American Medical Association's Principles of Medical Ethics make this commandment more specific; they prohibit a physician from revealing "confidences entrusted to him . . . or the deficiencies he may observe in the character of patients," except to the extent that disclosure is required by law or is necessary "to protect the welfare of the individual or of the community." In some states, the confidentiality of the doctor-patient relationship is reinforced by statutory prohibitions against the disclosure of certain types of information.

A distinction must be drawn between the physician-patient privilege and confidentiality. Most states have enacted statutes protecting patients from compulsory disclosure by their physicians in judicial proceedings of information about their diagnosis or treatment except where the patient waives the privilege. A physician's breach of this privilege could make him liable to the patient. The principle of confidentiality, on the other hand, applies to disclosures by the physician other than on the witness stand.[16]

It is clear that a physician has an ethical duty not to disclose confidential information concerning his patient, but the common law in the United States and England gave patients little protection.[17] In recent times, legislatures and courts have been more concerned to assure confidentiality. The cases in which a cause of action against a physician for damages has been recognized involve violation of a statute or violation of a patient-physician contract. For example, in *Munzer vs. Baisdell*[18] the plaintiff was awarded damages against the superintendent of a hospital for violation of a statute making all case records of a mental hospital confidential, except in circumstances not made out in that case. Generally, where the state licensure statute defines as misconduct the divulgence of a professional secret, violation may lead not only to revocation of the physician's license[19] but to civil liability in a suit brought by the patient.[20] Closely related to these cases are those in which courts have imposed liability on the theory that the contractual relationship between doctor and patient involves an implied agreement that information will be held in confidence.[21] In addition, if it is clear that the information revealed was intended to be kept private, an action against the disclosing physician might be based on the patient's right of privacy.[22] Moreover, if the information is false, the physician may be liable for libel or slander.[23]

The legal protection given to medical confidentiality is not absolute, however, and physicians may disclose information to proper persons for proper purposes. Where a statute requires a physician to report the existence of contagious or infectious diseases to a governmental body, the physician's compliance with this statute does not violate his duty of confidentiality to his patient.[24] Where the patient's communicable disease poses a great danger to others, the physician may also have the right, and indeed the duty, to inform them directly.[25] In the leading case of *Simonsen vs. Swenson,*[26] for example, the doctor was held not liable for informing the proprietress of the small hotel in which his patient was staying that the patient had a contagious disease.[27] Disclosure to the patient's spouse has generally been upheld even where the couple was separated[28] and where the physician expected the information would be used in a pending matrimonial suit.[29] It has been held that a physician may in good faith and with reasonable care convey information he believes to be true and to be necessary to protect a person outside the marriage partnership. In *Berry vs. Moench,*[30] it was held that a psychiatrist could properly disclose his patient's psychopathic personality to another physician who passed the information on to the parents of the patient's prospective bride.

The circumstances of the physician-patient relationship may themselves negate any implication of confidentiality. Thus, in *Hague vs. Williams,*[31] it was held that when parents applied for a life insurance policy on their child's life they lost the right to nondisclosure, and the physician was entitled to inform the insurance company, upon inquiry, that the child had a congenital heart condition. Similarly, when Dr. Geraci complied with the request of his patient's employer, the U.S. Air Force, to explain the underlying causes of illnesses he had previously certified and replied that the patient's absences were caused by alcoholism, the court held that he was permitted to make full disclosure. Since Dr. Geraci reasonably believed that the information was needed by the government, he was not liable to Mr. Clark.[32]

Accordingly, persons who undergo genetic screening in programs conducted by physicians would appear to have a legally protected right to have the screening results kept confidential in most American jurisdictions. This protection could be removed by a statute which required screeners to submit results to a state official. Physician-screeners may also enjoy a limited privilege to disclose the results of screening to third parties if necessary to enable them to protect themselves against seriously adverse consequences. It is difficult to say how far, if at all, this privilege will apply to genetic screening since the precedents all relate to disclosure concerning communicable diseases posing grave and immediate danger to the persons to whom disclosure is made. The presence of genetic conditions is obviously of a quite different character.

Again, it should be noted that the principle of confidentiality in genetic screening is based in part on the specific duty of physicians as professionals and the special physician-patient relationship. Therefore, one would expect that the principle would probably apply with less force when the screening is conducted outside of the physician-patient relationship. There are no precedents involving the confidentiality of information obtained concerning a person's health, mental or biologic characteristics, and the like, outside the physician-patient context. Whether a particular genetic screening program would be regarded as within or without such a relationship would turn upon the facts in that case. For instance, disclosure of information by a nonmedical screener might not be actionable in itself, but if his screening were performed in a hospital or medical clinic, a court might conclude that he is bound by the principle of confidentiality since his activities are subject to supervision by physicians. It may also appear that the screenee entertained the reasonable expectation that anyone who conducts genetic tests and has access to screening results – nurses, technicians or screening agencies, as well as physicians – will be bound by the same degree of secrecy and respect for privacy that underlies the screenee's original willingness to participate in such testing.[33]

Furthermore, a duty of confidentiality on the part of nonphysicians may follow upon statutory recognition that they are engaged in a profession and subjected to licensure. For example, a number of states have enacted statutes requiring licensure of psychologists and providing for a psychologist-client privilege.[34] Although no cases involving psychologists have been found, it may be expected that a corollary of their statutory status will be the emergence of a duty of confidentiality akin to that of the physician, with liability to the patient for breach of the duty.

Thus, under existing law, it cannot be said with certainty that the results of genetic screening must always be held in the same degree of confidence that governs the doctor-patient relationship. Screening agencies should, of course, proceed on the presumption that data may not be communicated to persons other than the one screened, since any deviation from this principle exposes the agency to the risk of liability. But there are exceptions to the principle of confidentiality, and the screening agency will have to determine in each instance whether or not any proposed disclosure to other parties falls within one of these exceptions.

Results of Screening Conducted Without Specific Consent

A special case is presented by the possibility that physicians and hospitals may undertake genetic screening on a routine basis without the specific consent of the patient. While this would not fall within the category of a strictly voluntary screening program, it is appropriate to discuss it here since it would probably be performed by persons associated with voluntary programs, rather than by mandatory state-sponsored programs. The justification offered for screening without specific consent would probably be the general rule that when a patient places himself in the hands of a physician, relying entirely upon the experience and skill of the physician, he gives implied consent to whatever action the physician reasonably believes is necessary. Thus, where genetic screening is relevant to the purpose for which the patient has sought diagnosis or treatment, such screening would be proper under the implied consent rule and would, in a sense, be voluntary. It is highly doubtful, however, that implied consent to genetic screening would be found where, for example, the patient was being treated for a broken leg, or where the screening was for research or statistical purposes. In such cases the screening would clearly be involuntary and would expose the screener to liability for assault and battery.[35]

Where the screening is without specific consent, but is voluntary under the implied consent doctrine, the principles on disclosure and confidentiality set forth in the preceding subsections would apply. Since the patient may be unaware that he has been screened, it is unlikely that he will press his physician for the test results. Yet his unawareness should only serve to increase the physician's obligations to take care in informing the patient and in protecting his privacy, since the screening occurred because of the patient's complete trust in the physician and cooperation in the tests he prescribed.

In cases of involuntary screening, the physician would certainly be held to a duty of confidentiality at least as great as that in voluntary screening programs. The problem of disclosure of the information to the patient is, however, much more complex, and has not been resolved by the courts. On the one hand, it can be forcefully argued that the physician has a duty to disclose the information to the patient, particularly if the information could be of benefit to him. On the other hand, the patient's receipt of unsolicited and unexpected information that he has or is a carrier of a genetic disorder could have an unsettling, and perhaps injurious, effect which might justify imposition of liability on the physician. That potential ought to give screeners further pause before they attempt to test persons without their knowledge and consent, express or implied.

Screening by Public Agencies

The discussion of the problems of disclosure and confidentiality with respect to private screening programs apply with equal force to screening programs conducted by public agencies. Moreover, the confidentiality of public health records is required by statute in some states and such statutes would, of course, enhance the protection given to records of genetic screening undertaken by a public body.

Voluntary genetic screening programs conducted by public agencies do, however, involve one unique aspect – that is, the possibility that such a program may run afoul of constitutional prohibitions. At least to the extent relevant to genetic screening, the constitutional prohibitions involved apply only to actions of state and federal governments. Of course, a screening program financed in whole or in part by governmental funds might be regarded as "state action" subject to constitutional limitations though conducted by a "private" agency.

Since voluntary genetic screening programs conducted or funded by public agencies involve no compulsion and do not impose burdens or deprivations on unwilling persons, the range of relevant constitutional considerations is sharply limited. The only constitutional issue which might reasonably arise would be whether the equal protection clause of the Fourteenth Amendment forbids making genetic screening available only to specified groups. If, for example a public agency were to provide screening services only to blacks for sickle cell anemia or only to

Ashkenazi Jews for Tay-Sachs disease, it could be argued that such a program is discriminatory in the sense that it singles out specified groups for the receipt of government-granted benefits.

The equal protection clause does not require that all persons must be given the same benefits by the law or that all similar problems must be dealt with at one time[36]; "there is no constitutional requirement that a regulation, in other respects permissible, must reach every class to which it might be applied – that the Legislature must be held rigidly to the choice of regulating all or none."[37] The government may, for example, fluoridate public water supplies to minimize dental caries without having at the same time to provide free flu shots. Legislatures are permitted to draw distinctions and to construct classifications.[38] For a classification to survive attack under the equal protection clause it must be based on differences that are rationally related to the purposes for which it was made[39] and must not work an invidious discrimination.[40] The legislators may provide public housing for poor people without providing public housing for rich people. Similarly, they may attack the problem of sickle cell anemia without attacking the problem of Cooley anemia if there exist any reasonable bases on which to distinguish these diseases from each other and from other disorders that are similar in having a genetic origin.

A classification based on race or religion, however, is inherently suspect, whether explicit or *de facto,* and the government has the burden of justifying such a classification.[41] Thus, while a governmental program to screen only for sickle cell anemia – a "black disease" – would not violate equal protection, a statute specifying that only blacks could be screened by a public agency would probably be unconstitutional, since non-black persons may also carry the sickle cell gene. If, however, sickle cell screening were made available to all persons "at risk," there would probably be no violation of equal protection if only blacks in fact came in to be screened. If a white person who presented himself were denied screening on the ground that he was not "at risk," the constitutionality of the denial would depend on whether the determination of "risk" was "reasonable" in a Fourteenth Amendment sense.[42]

Compulsory Genetic Screening

Different questions are raised by mandatory genetic screening programs pursuant to statutes prescribing the testing of everyone, or of specific classes of individuals, with penalties or deprivation of benefits for those who refuse to submit to screening. For example, most states presently require screening of newborn infants for phenylketonuria (PKU), an inborn error of metabolism which usually causes mental retardation if not treated early in life. At present some states and the District of Columbia require screening for sickle cell anemia and sickle cell trait for all school children and attempts will doubtless be made before long to go beyond sickle cell disease and require screening for certain genetic conditions and carrier states as a prerequisite to obtaining a marriage license.[43]

Questions have been raised as to whether such genetic screening programs may be unlawful on constitutional grounds, a matter which has never been decided by the courts. Two separate issues are thus presented: (1) whether the legislature has the power to enact compulsory screening measures, and (2) whether, if the power exists, its exercise violates any constitutional prohibitions.

The Power to Promote Public Health Through Genetic Screening

Power of the Federal Government. The powers exercisable by the federal government are limited to those enumerated in the Constitution,[44] which does not give Congress any express power to legislate with respect to the public health and welfare. Congress does, however, have the power to enact legislation dealing with the public health as an incident to its explicit powers, for example, to regulate commerce or to provide for the national defense. It is likely that a mandatory genetic screening statute enacted by Congress would be found by the courts to come within the greatly expanded scope of federal authority (primarily under the commerce clause) that has been recognized in the last few decades. This is probably only a hypothetic possibility, since Congress has not been disposed to enact legislation of this kind which would impinge upon an area that traditionally has been regarded as within the power of the states. Congress does, nevertheless, have direct power to enact health legislation to certain limited areas which are within the scope of its authority, such as the District of Columbia, federal employment or the armed services.

Power of the States. Under the Constitution of the United States, exercise of police power (ie the power to take action to protect and promote the health, welfare and safety of the public) rests in the first instance with the states. "The range of state power is not defined and delimited by an enumeration of legislative subject-matter"[45] in the United States Constitution. Rather, the scope of the police power of any state is defined and limited by the state's own constitution. Since there is great variation in state constitutions, no useful purpose would be served by attempting to analyze them here in order to determine whether genetic screening would be encompassed by the police power of particular states. This would be a matter for decision by the legislators, and if necessary the judges, of each state.

Relationship to a Valid Governmental Purpose. This is not to say that the Constitution of the United States has no bearing on whether a public health measure promulgated by a state (or by federal authorities regarding the District of Columbia) is a valid exercise of the police power. The government may prescribe reasonable regulations in order to protect or promote the health, safety, morals and welfare of the community,[46] but under the Fifth and Fourteenth Amendments to the Constitution any such regulations must be reasonably related to a legitimate state purpose.[47] The threshold question, then, is whether compulsory genetic screening programs would be open to challenge for failing to foster a permissible end that may be sought by the government.

Like the numerous public health measures on the books in every state, a genetic screening program might be expected to serve a number of purposes, including: (1) the provision of information about the incidence and severity of the disease; (2) the protection of members of the public from disease; and (3) the conservation of health resources through the prevention and appropriate treatment of disease. As long as plausible justifications for screening such as these can be found, it is unlikely that the judiciary would seriously entertain a challenge to a screening program on the ground that it lacked efficacy in promoting legitimate state purposes.

At one time in American constitutional history, the Supreme Court undertook to strike down public health legislation when it concluded that the legislation did not comport with "due process" under the Fifth and Fourteenth Amendments. The high point of this stance was the case of *Lochner vs. New York,*[48] where a New York statute limiting the hours of work of bakery employees was declared unconstitutional. The Supreme Court held that the ordinance could not be justified as a public health measure but was rather an attempt to regulate in the economic sphere, by limiting the freedom of bakery owners and bakery employees to contract with each other. The issue, as the Court saw it, was:

> "Is this a fair, reasonable, and appropriate exercise of the police power of the state, or is it an unreasonable, unnecessary, and arbitrary interference with the right of the individual to his personal liberty or to enter into those contracts in relation to labor which seem to him appropriate or necessary for the support of himself and his family?"[49]

The Court concluded that there was "no reasonable foundation for holding this to be necessary or appropriate as a health law to safeguard the public health, or the health of the individuals who are following the trade of a baker."[50]

After *Lochner,* the Supreme Court gradually adopted a more liberal view of governmental authority and ceased substituting its own judgment for that of legislatures on the wisdom and necessity of such economic legislation, and by the mid-1930s it had backed off entirely from its "substantive due process" position. It is now generally accepted that a legislature has no burden to justify the reasonableness of or need for such a regulation; rather, the burden of demonstrating that it is not a valid exercise of the police power rests with the party attacking the statute. A statute will not be declared unconstitutional "unless in the light of facts made known or generally assumed it is of such a character as to preclude the assumption that it rests upon some rational basis within the knowledge or experience of the legislators."[51]

Accordingly, it is highly unlikely that a mandatory genetic screening statute would be held unconstitutional on the ground that it is unnecessary or unwise, if it appears that there is any rational relationship between its effects and a legitimate governmental purpose. This would be the case even if the genetic conditions discovered as a result of screening were not amenable to treatment. The Supreme Court would probably conclude that there was a rational basis for the statute in that the legislators may have had in mind the other kinds of benefits suggested previously, such as information about incidence and severity of the disease, a reduction in the number of affected children born, and a consequent conservation of health resources. In other words, under the present state of constitutional law, it is not likely that the judiciary would second guess the legislature as to the usefulness of a compulsory genetic screening program.

Constitutional Limitations on Governmental Action

Putting aside the question of governmental power, then, the validity of a compulsory genetic screening program will depend primarily on whether it impinges impermissibly upon individual rights protected by the United States Constitution.[52] In recent years, the courts have elaborated a number of areas in which they apply special scrutiny to the actions of the legislative and executive branches. While judges no longer use the due process clause to strike down economic legislation which they believe to be unwise or unnecessary, other kinds of state action that encroach on personal liberty – especially on so-called fundamental rights – are increasingly found to run afoul of the Constitution.[53] Moreover, neither state nor federal authorities may deny citizens the "equal protection of the laws."[54] Both of these constitutional limitations are relevant in analyzing compulsory genetic screening programs.

Due Process and Fundamental Rights. In recent years the Supreme Court has identified certain rights as "fundamental" ones, interference with which requires greater justification. Although not all constitutionally guaranteed rights are regarded as fundamental, some of the fundamental rights are those specifically protected by the Constitution, such as freedom of religion and of speech.[55] In other cases, the Court has found fundamental rights not explicitly mentioned in the Constitution, such as the right of privacy[56] which has recently been held to include the right to make certain decisions about health care free of certain restrictions.[57] A law which restricts those liberties that are "so rooted in the traditions and conscience of our people as to be ranked as fundamental,"[58] is subject to specially rigorous examination as to whether it violates the due process clause. Legislation impinging on such a right must be supported by a heavy burden of justification going far beyond the usual "rational basis" test. The state must show at least that the governmental objective or classification[59] is supported by a compelling interest and that no alternative means, with lesser impingement on these rights, are available for accomplishment of that objective. Indeed, in some cases, the Supreme Court has held that certain activities, within the scope of the fundamental rights, are totally beyond the power of government to regulate.[60]

Among the fundamental rights there are two groups associated with the constitutional right of privacy which have particular relevance to genetic screening: those rights relating to marriage and procreation and those concerning a person's control of his or her own body.

For some time the Supreme Court has given explicit recognition to the rights which protect decisions about one's family.[61] Marriage itself has been termed "fundamental to our very existence and survival"[62] and "one of the basic civil rights of man."[63] Free decisionmaking about procreation is also recognized as a fundamental right.[64] Indeed, it was in the context of state regulation of procreation that the "right of privacy" received forceful articulation in the landmark case of *Griswold vs. Connecticut.*[65] In that case, the Supreme Court held unconstitutional a statute making the use of, or assistance in the use of, contraceptives a crime. In reaching this conclusion, the Court found a fundamental "right of privacy older than the Bill of Rights,"[66] and though not mentioned therein still established by the "penumbras" surrounding the First, Fourth, Fifth, Sixth, and Ninth Amendments to the Constitution.[67] The Court held that the marital relationship falls within a constitutionally protected zone of privacy and that the law prohibiting *use* of contraceptives has a "maximum destructive impact"[68] on that relationship. Yet it must be remembered that the decision did not go so far as to declare that married couples have an absolute right to use contraceptives, since the Court suggested that a statute prohibiting manufacture or sale of contraceptives might be constitutional.

The constitutionally protected zone of privacy was extended in *Eisenstadt vs. Baird*[69] to decisions about childbearing by unmarried as well as married persons. Baird had been convicted under a Massachusetts statute prohibiting the distribution of contraceptives to unmarried persons, and the Court affirmed a discharge of his conviction on the ground that there was no rational basis for the separate classification of unmarried persons. In so doing, the Court made clear the fundamental nature of the right at issue: "If the right of privacy means anything, it is the right of the *individual*, married or single, to be free from unwarranted govermmental intrusion into matters so fundamentally affecting a person as the decision whether to bear or beget a child."[70]

In *Roe vs. Wade*[71] the zone of privacy was found to be "broad enough to encompass a woman's decision whether or not to terminate her pregnancy."[72] The Supreme Court ruled, however, that the right to choose an abortion is not unqualified and must be weighed against the state's interests in protecting the health of pregnant women and in safeguarding potential life. "These interests are separate and distinct. Each grows in substantiality as the woman approaches term and, at a point during pregnancy,, each becomes 'compelling'."[73] Since abortion during the first trimester is safer for a woman than continuing her pregnancy to term, the Court held that the decision to abort during this period lies with the woman and her physician, "free of interference by the State."[74] During the second trimester the qualifications of persons performing abortions, the places where they are performed, and so forth, may be regulated to promote the safety of the procedure. During the final trimester, once the fetus is "viable," the state "may, if it chooses, regulate, and even proscribe, abortion except where it is necessary, in appropriate medical judgment, for the preservation of the life or health of the mother."[75]

A number of the major purposes which the state might have in mandating genetic screening, such as preventing disease and saving state resources, are obviously based on the expected connection between screening results and decisions about marriage and procreation. In light of the cases, the question must be confronted whether it is permissible for the state to compel genetic screening for these purposes. This is a problem which has not yet been resolved by the courts. If screening were linked by statute with restrictions on marriage and procreation (eg mandatory abortion) or were conducted in such a way as to coerce screenees' decisions on these matters, it would probably be found invalid under the *Griswold* line of cases. It is likely, however, that any restrictions placed on marriage and procreation that would result from genetic screening would be only indirect – that is, the result of choices made by individuals in consequence of the information about themselves brought to their attention by the state. Screening results presented in a noncoercive fashion would probably be comparable to such permissible state activities as sex education classes. Moreover, some restrictions on marriage are permissible; for example, most states already prohibit marriage between persons of a stated degree of relationship. To the extent that such legislation can be justified on genetic grounds,[76] it has yet to be judged in light of post-*Griswold* jurisprudence on marriage-related decisions. This also raises the issue of whether, and how, the state may infringe on one person's liberty to protect another person or the community in general.

One is thus brought to the second aspect of "privacy" which may be relevant to compulsory genetic screening – control over one's own body. As was already suggested, this issue was raised in *Roe,* but in a slightly different context. There the question was whether the state could limit potentially risky but voluntary activities, while in genetic screening the question is whether the individual can limit the state's interference with his or her body by asserting, as Justice Brandeis once wrote, a "right to be let alone – the most comprehensive of rights and the right most valued by civilized men."[77] The Supreme Court did not have to decide that issue in *Roe,* and the Justices felt that it was "not clear" whether the absolute right claimed by some "to do with one's body as one pleases bears a close relationship to the right of privacy."[78] Mr. Justice Blackmun cited two cases to illustrate that the Supreme Court has not found such an absolute right.

The first was *Jacobson vs. Massachusetts,*[79] which upheld the conviction of a man who had refused to submit to compulsory smallpox vaccination during an epidemic in Cambridge. He offered to prove that he had been made seriously ill when vaccinated as a child and that there was no way to determine "with any degree of certainty"[80] whether one's blood was in such a condition as to render vaccination dangerous. This evidence was excluded by the trial court as immaterial, and the Supreme Court affirmed on the ground that the offers of proof invited the court improperly "to go over the whole ground gone over by the legislature when it enacted the statute in question."[81] *Jacobson* would thus seem neither to condemn nor to sanction legislation mandating genetic screening. On the one hand, it appears that the immediate physical risks of the procedure to the screenee would be so slight as not to justify interfering with the legislative judgment. On the other hand, the state's interest in seeing that screening is done seems much less compelling than in the stemming of an epidemic. While the interference with the person is small, it may be resisted if no interference at all is justified, as Justice Harlan stated in *Jacobson*:

> There is . . . a sphere within which the individual may assert the supremacy of his own will and rightfully dispute the authority of any human government, especially of any free government existing under a written constitution, to interfere with the exercise of that will. But it is equally true that in every well-ordered society charged with the duty of conserving the safety of its members the rights of the individual in respect of his liberty may at times, under the pressure of great dangers, be subjected to such restraint, to be enforced by reasonable regulations, as the safety of the general public may demand.[82]

Jacobson thus speaks in terms of protecting others from "great dangers," an apt description of the consequences of many genetic diseases. This concern for the health of future generations is a legitimate one which is also exemplified in the laws restricting marriage to those who have passed an examination for veneral disease.[83] Yet it must be read in the context of the more recent cases such as *Griswold* and *Roe* that exhibit a greater concern for privacy and bodily integrity.

Although the interference sanctioned in *Jacobson* not only served a pressing public need but involved a minimal intrusion, a much greater invasion of privacy – and interference with the right to procreate – was upheld in *Buck vs. Bell,*[84] the second case cited by Mr. Justice Blackmun in *Roe.* At issue in *Buck* was a Virginia statute authorizing the sterilization of institutionalized "feeble minded" persons. The Supreme Court upheld the law against a due process challenge, stating that it would be better if society, rather than having to wait for the misdeeds or destitution of feeble-minded persons' feeble-minded offspring, could instead "prevent those who are manifestly unfit from continuing their kind."[85]

In the nearly 50 years since *Buck* was decided there have been great changes in geneticists' confidence in making sweeping characterizations of "manifest unfitness." Indeed, the increased sophistication of genetics and its ability to identify the inheritance of many more disorders, makes the medical model underlying the compulsory sterilization of "imbeciles" seem terrifyingly naive. It is doubtful that any court would accept compulsory sterilization for any of a host of genetic diseases for which carrier screening is now possible – many of them far worse conditions than feeble-mindedness – simply on the authority of *Buck vs. Bell.*

The past half century has wrought changes not only in genetic knowledge but in the law's attitude toward state infringements on basic rights. In *Skinner vs. Oklahoma,*[86] which was decided on equal protection grounds without having to reach the due process argument, the Court manifested a very different attitude toward compulsory sterilization:

> We are dealing here with legislation which involves one of the basic civil rights of man. Marriage and procreation are fundamental to the very existence and survival of the race. The power to sterilize, if exercised, may have subtle, far-reaching and devastating effects. In evil or reckless hands it can cause races or types which are inimical to the dominant group to wither and disappear. There is no redemption for the individual whom the law touches. Any experiment which the State conducts is to his irreparable injury. He is forever deprived of a basic liberty.[87]

Yet *Skinner* did not overrule *Buck* and the latter's recent citation in *Roe* means that it must be examined seriously.

The Supreme Court affirmed the state court's decision in *Buck,* which rested on two grounds for permitting involuntary sterilization. The primary reason was to promote the health and welfare of the patient. Without sterilization she might involuntarily bear another illegitimate child; with sterilization she could "be discharged with safety [from the institution] and become self-supporting."[88] *Buck,* like *Roe,* thus lends some support to genetic screening intended to protect the screenee's own health or welfare – as where, for example, screening could reveal a late-onset disease which could be prevented or ameliorated through early detection and treatment. It is well to keep in mind, however, the factual background of these cases: in *Buck* the alternative to sterilization was a lifetime in the "State Colony for Epileptics and Feeble Minded" with the constant risk of repeated unwanted pregnancies, and in *Roe* the Court spoke approvingly of the state's interest in safeguarding life and health not in terms of state action to promote better health but only to keep people from engaging in life-threatening conduct (unsafe, nonmedical abortions). Unless the genetic disorder were severe and the means were at hand to prevent its manifestation, compulsory screening would not be justified under this branch of the reasoning in Buck.[89]

The second reason for the *Buck* decision flows from the first: Carrie Buck's sterilization and release were predicted to save the state money, both for her maintenance and for that of any offspring in need of institutional care. *Buck* would thus appear to validate screening designed to reduce health expenditures. Yet the Supreme Court has recently made clear that a potential saving in state funds, or even a requirement to expend them, is not sufficient grounds for the abridgement of fundamental constitutional rights or for the drawing of an invidious classification.[90] It remains to be seen how the Court would weigh the state's financial interests against the claim that mandatory genetic screening violates a right of privacy or of bodily integrity.

Accordingly, while the present state of constitutional law does not provide a definite answer about the validity of compulsory genetic screening, no case stands either as a clear bar to, or an unequivocal precedent for, such a government effort. Clearly, a definite gap remains between the Supreme Court's decisions on "fundamental rights" and the burdens that may be imposed by mandatory genetic screening. This gap can probably best be bridged by legislation assuring that any such screening programs will not unduly infringe on the privacy or self-determination of the people screened.

This analysis is limited, however, to the kinds of mandatory genetic screening programs now in existence. Other kinds of genetic screening, – for example, mandatory amniocentesis – would raise more difficult constitutional questions because of the greater burdens and risks involved to the subjects – factors which entered into both the *Jacobson* and *Roe* decisions – because mandatory amniocentesis may in fact approach mandatory abortion. Mandatory counseling and abortion or explicit restrictions on marriage resulting from mandatory screening would probably run afoul of the *Griswold* doctrine. In addition, the uses to which information resulting from mandatory genetic screening is put may raise new, substantial constitutional problems. The use of the results of mandatory screening for purposes of subsequently classifying individuals for special treatment, – for example, the classification of XYY males for special education or the use of information for insurance or occupational purposes, – might infringe constitutional rights.

Equal Protection. If a compulsory genetic screening program were to single out a particular class of persons for screening, members of the class might challenge the program on the ground that it imposed a discriminatory burden on them in violation of the equal protection clause. Although the problem of classification does not admit of "doctrinaire definition,"[91] a classification will be upheld if it can be concluded that the classification is reasonably related to a legitimate purpose of the state.[92] For example, a state may single out the class of persons who handle food in restaurants for mandatory chest x rays or other forms of screening.

In recent years, however, the Supreme Court has announced a new and more stringent test applicable in equal protection cases where statutes involve classifications which are "constitutionally suspect." Where the classification is drawn on racial, religious or ethnic lines, it is regarded as inherently suspect and a more stringent test is applied. This trend is illustrated in two recent Supreme Court decisions involving laws prohibiting miscegenation. In *McLaughlin vs. Florida*[93] the Court held that racial classifications are "conditionally suspect" and that such a classification will be upheld "only if it is necessary, and not merely rationally related, to the accomplishment of a permissible state policy."[94] In the second case, *Loving vs. Virginia,*[95] the Court explicitly rejected the rational basis test in favor of imposing a "very heavy burden of justification" on the state.

Accordingly, if a statute singles out blacks for mandatory sickle cell screening, Jews for Tay-Sachs screening or persons of Mediterranean descent for Cooley anemia screening, this would, presumably, involve a "suspect" classification imposing a heavy burden of justification, perhaps even a showing of necessity, upon the state. If the program were regarded as essentially beneficial and if the burdens were regarded as minimal, the stringency of the test might be reduced.[96]

Conclusion

Genetic screening programs should be conducted on the principles that results of the screening will be communicated to the persons screened and to no other person. If the screenee is (implicitly or explicitly) promised the diagnosis, the screener will be liable for failure to convey it to him. Otherwise, disclosure may be required under the law governing the physician-patient relationship, but whether this is required by law would depend on the details of the screening program. The requirement of confidentiality is also found in common law precedents arising out of the physician-patient relationship and in statutory law on professional standards for licensure. This requirement would be enforceable in a civil proceeding initiated by a screenee who was injured by breach of confidentiality. The law also recognizes exceptions to these principles, although any deviation would have to be justified by the screening agency.

Government screening programs conducted on a voluntary basis do not seem to involve any insurmountable constitutional problems. Compulsory screening programs are probably within the public health powers of the states if they serve any of a number of legitimate governmental purposes such as supplying research data, diminishing harm to future generations or saving resources. If compulsory screening is applicable to members of specified racial, religious or ethnic groups, it would have to meet a heavy burden of justification, and a violation of the equal protection clause of the Fourteenth Amendment may be found. Compulsory screening may also interfere with a number of fundamental rights, centering on the constitutional right of privacy. Existing case law does not, however, resolve the questions thus presented. In the present state of constitutional law, it is not possible to predict whether a screening program would be held to violate any fundamental constitutionally protected rights. It can be said that it is not clearly ruled out by any decided case, while it is also admitted that a number of older cases which seem to support compulsory screening were decided when the state of the art – both genetic and legal – was fundamentally different than it is today.

Footnotes

1. Screening of adults for carrier status may lead to amniocentesis in carrier-carrier pregnancies (if the genetic disease is diagnosable prenatally) and in turn to the abortion of affected fetuses; amniocentesis itself can also be considered a type of screening. Legislators who oppose abortion might thus be tempted to place limits on screening and amniocentesis. Such efforts would clearly run afoul of *Roe vs. Wade,* 410 U.S. 113, 1973, which not only established a woman's almost unfettered right to undergo a medically-supervised abortion until the point of fetal viability, but also made clear that the state's authority to interfere with any decisions about medical care is severely limited by the individual's constitutional "right of privacy."
2. The term "diagnosis" is used here in the context of the results of the screening procedure; these may either be a firm diagnosis or, more likely, an indication that the individual appears to have or to be a carrier of the genetic condition being screened for, and that further tests should be conducted to establish a definite diagnosis.
3. In this paper, the terms "screenee" and "person screened" include any person, such as a parent, guardian, or other designee (such as the physician) of the person actually screened, who would be deemed his legal representative or who was specially designated for this purpose.
4. Other kinds of cases can be visualized. For example, a case in which the screening agency accidentally injures the screenee in the process of performing the tests, or where the screening agency gives false information to third parties. Such cases do not, however, involve unusual legal issues and would be resolved on the basis of the laws of negligence, defamation, etc. For a discussion of the potential liability of screening programs for errors in the choice of the screening procedure, the execution of that procedure and the notification of test results,

see Franklin, *Medical Mass Screening Programs: A Legal Appraisal* 47 CORNELL L. Q. 205 (1962).

5. RESTATEMENT OF CONTRACTS § §329 (compensatory damages for substantial injury) and 330 (foreseeability of harm as a requisite for recovery); cf. § 345 (damages for breach of contract for the benefit of a third person) (1932). See also RESTATEMENT OF TORTS SECOND § §323(b) (negligent performance of services causing harm because plaintiff relies on defendant's undertaking), 324A(c) (same, where injury occurs to third person).
6. RESTATEMENT OF CONTRACTS §90 (promise reasonably inducing definite and substantial action).
7. *Stafford vs. Shultz,* 42 Cal. 2d 767, 270 P. 2d 1 (1954); *Berkey vs. Anderson,* 1 Cal. App. 3d 790, 82 Cal. Rptr. 67 (1969). The scope of the physician's duty is limited, of course, to information generally relating to the reasons for which he was consulted.
8. See eg, *Canterbury vs. Spence,* 464 F. 2d 772 (D. C. Cir. 1972); *Natanson vs. Kline,* 186 Kans. 393, 350 P. 2d 1093, *clarified and rehearing denied,* 187 Kans. 186, 354 P. 2d 670 (1960); *Salgo vs. Leland Stanford University,* 154 Cal. App. 2d 560, 317 P. 2d 170 (1957).
9. *Canterbury vs. Spence,* 464 F. 2d 772, 781 (D. C. Cir. 1972).
10. See eg, *Lester vs. Aetna Casualty & Surety Co.,* 240 F. 2d 676 (5th Cir. 1957); *Hunt vs. Bradshaw* 242 N. C. 517, 88 S. E. 2d 762 (1955).
11. *Cobbs vs. Grant,* 104 Cal. Rptr. 505, 502 P. 2d 1 (1972); *Wilkinson vs. Vesey,* 295 A. 2d 676 (R. I. 1972); *Canterbury vs. Spence,* 464 F 2d 772 (D. C. Cir. 1972).
12. *Cobbs vs. Grant,* 104 Cal. Rptr. 505, 516, 502 P. 2d 1, 12 (1972).
13. *Dowling vs. Mutual Life Ins. Co.,* 168 So. 2d 107 (La. App. 1964), *writ refused,* 247 La. 248, 170 So. 2d 508 (1965) (*held*, physician had duty to warn patient that x ray indicated need of further tests for more accurate diagnosis); *Doty vs. Lutheran Hosp. Ass'n,* 110 Neb. 467, 194 N. W. 444 (1923) (*held*, error to direct verdict for defendant physician when evidence showed that physician failed to inform patient that he had smallpox at time of discharge from hospital). Cf. *Tvedt vs. Haugen,* 70 N. D. 338, 294 N. W. 183, 188 (1940) (Judgment for patient affirmed: "Plaintiff's leg was not getting along fine, but quite the contrary. Defendant must have known, or should have known, that there was something wrong about it. He did not inform the plaintiff as to his true condition."); *Dietze vs. King,* 184 F. Supp. 944 (E. D. Va. 1960) (judgment for patient where physician withheld his belief that he had left sponge in her during operation).
14. *Union Carbide & Carbon Corp. vs. Stapleton,* 237 F. 2d 229 (6th Cir. 1956) (affirming judgment for employee against employer for failure to inform employee of his tubercular condition disclosed by employer's medical examination); *Wojcik vs. Aluminum Co. of America,* 18 Misc. 2d 740, 183 N. Y. S. 2d 35 (Sup. Ct. 1959) (*held,* plaintiff's allegation that he relied on defendant to inform him of any irregularities revealed by medical examination conducted by defendant's physicians and that defendant failed to inform him of developing tuberculosis, states a cause of action in tort independent of Workmen's Compensation Law).

15. *Union Carbide & Carbon Corp. vs. Stapleton,* 237 F. 2d 229, 232 (6th Cir. 1956). The cases declare liability where the failure to inform is negligent or intentional.
16. The adoption in most states of an explicit privilege to exclude courtroom revelations but not extrajudicial disclosures is explained by the fact that "because of the high ethical standards of the medical profession, very few cases of extrajudicial disclosures arise, whereas physicians are frequently requested to testify in court." Note, 79 HARV. L. REV. 1723, 1724 (1966). See also DeWitt, *Medical Ethics and the Law: The Conflict Between Dual Allegiances,* 5 WEST. RES. L. REV. 5, 19 (1953).
17. An action would lie at common law where the communication amounted to a libel or slander. *AB vs. CD,* 14 Sess. Cas. (Dunlop) 2d ser. 177 (1851).
18. 49 N. Y. S. 2d 915 (Sup. Ct. 1944).
19. See eg, *McPheeters vs. Bd. of Medical Examiners,* 103 Cal. App. 297, 284 P. 938 (1930). *McPheeters* holds that to prove a "willful betraying of a professional secret" a deliberate act done with a wrongful purpose must be shown; it was not found in that case, since no patient complained about the information conveyed by Dr. McPheeters to his former office assistant.
20. See eg, *Simonsen vs. Swenson,* 104 Neb. 224, 177 N. W. 831 (1920); *Hammonds vs. Aetna Casualty & Surety Co.,* 237 F. Supp. 96 (N. D. Ohio 1965). But see *Quarles vs. Sutherland,* 215 Tenn. 651, 389 S. W. 2d 249 (1965). In *Simonsen,* the court held that although a civil action would lie for a wrongful breach of the statute, none occurred where the physician believed the plaintiff to be infected with a contagious disease and disclosed this to those who were in danger of being infected. "A disclosure in such case would ... not be a betrayal of the confidence of the patient, since the patient must know . . . that, in the exception stated, his disease may be disclosed." 104 Neb. at 228-229, 177 N. W. at 832.
21. See eg, *Barry vs. Moench,* 8 Utah 2d 191, 331 P. 2d 814 (1958); *Smith vs. Driscoll,* 94 Wash. 441, 162 P. 572 (1917); *Clark vs. Geraci,* 29 Misc. 2d 791, 794, 208 N. Y. S. 2d 564, 567 (Sup. Ct. 1960) (cause of action "is implied by our statutory law and widely conceived in the doctor-patient relationship"). Cf. *Alexander vs. Knight,* 197 Pa. Super. 79, 177 A. 2d 142, 146 (1962) (physician's breach of confidential relationship with plaintiff condemmed) (dictum).
22. See generally PROSSER, TORTS § 117 (4th ed. 1971); Note, *Medical Practice and the Right to Privacy,* 43 MINN. L. REV. 943 (1959).
23. *Berry vs. Moench,* 8 Utah 2d 191, 331 P. 2d 814 (1958), was a libel action against a physician who disclosed allegedly "false and derogatory information" about his former patient's mental condition to the physician of the patient's prospective bride. The Utah Supreme Court even suggested that liability might be found for even true statements, since information resulting from a physician-patient relationship is likely to be embarrassing to the patient if revealed. See note 17 supra.
24. DeWitt, supra note 16, at 8. In some states, statutes specifically protect from civil liability to his patient any physician who makes such disclosures in good faith, eg, MINN. STAT. ANN. § 144.68 (1970); OHIO REV. CODE § 4731.22 (1953).
25. *Davis vs. Rodman,* 147 Ark. 385, 227 S. W. 612 (1921) (defendant physicians, who did not advise either board of health or members of family that two

children under their care had typhoid fever, held not liable for resulting injuries to other family members only because plaintiffs failed to allege that defendants' negligence was proximate cause of injuries); *Medlin vs. Bloom*, 230 Mass. 201, 119 N. E. 773 (1918) (whether physician's failure promptly to notify board of health of plaintiff's condition caused plaintiff's blindness was a question for the jury).

26. 104 Neb. 224, 117 N. W. 831 (1920).
27. The testimony at trial showed that there was "much danger of [the plaintiff] communicating the disease [syphilis] to others in the hotel," since it "is very readily transmitted in its early stages, and could be carried through drinking cups, eating utensils, and other articles handled or used by the diseased person." Id. at 225-226, 177 N. W. at 831.
28. *Pennision vs. Provident Life & Acc. Ins. Co.*, 154 So. 2d 617 (La. App. 1963).
29. *Curry vs. Corn*, 277 N. Y. S. 2d 470 (1966).
30. 8 Utah 2d 191, 331 P. 2d 814 (1958).
31. 37 N. J. 328, 181 A. 2d 345 (1962).
32. *Clark vs. Geraci*, 29 Misc. 2d 791, 208 N. Y. S. 2d 564 (Sup. Ct. 1960).
33. Cf. *Barber vs. Time, Inc.*, 348 Mo. 1199, 159 S. W. 2d 291 (1942).
34. See Fischer, *The Psychotherapeutic Professions and the Law of Privileged Communications*, 10 WAYNE L. REV. 609, 638 (1964).
35. Eg, *Hively vs. Higgs*, 120 Ore. 588, 253 P. 363 (1927); *Schloendorff vs. Society of New York Hospital*, 211 N. Y. 125, 105 N. E. 92 (1914). Also see the recent cases on "informed consent," note 8 supra.
36. *Richardson vs. Belcher*, 404 U. S. 78 (1971); *A. F. of L. vs. American Sash & Door Co.*, 335 U. S. 538 (1949); *Semler vs. Oregon State Bd. of Dental Examiners*, 294 U. S. 608 (1935). But see *Shapiro vs. Thompson*, 394 U. S. 618, 632-33 (1969) (benefits may not be differentiated on basis of recipient's past tax contributions to state).
37. *Silver vs. Silver*, 280 U. S. 117, 123 (1929); accord, *Williamson vs. Lee Optical Co.*, 348 U. S. 483, 489 (1955); *West Coast Hotel Co. vs. Parrish*, 300 U. S. 379, 400 (1937).
38. *Railway Express Agency vs. New York*, 336 U. S. 106 (1949); *Tigner vs. Texas*, 310 U. S. 141 (1940).
39. *Morey vs. Doud*, 354 U. S. 457 (1957); *Smith vs. Cahoon*, 283 U. S. 553 (1931).
40. *Dandridge vs. Williams*, 397 U. S. 471 (1969); *Williamson vs. Lee Optical Co.*, 348 U. S. 483 (1955).
41. *Loving vs. Virginia*, 388 U. S. 1 (1967); *Korematsu vs. United States*, 323 U. S. 214 (1944).
42. See eg, *Levey vs. Louisiana*, 391 U. S. 68 (1968) (classification unreasonable); *McGowan vs. Maryland*, 366 U. S. 420, 1961 (classification reasonable); *Mayflower Farms vs. Ten Eyck*, 297 U. S. 266, 1936 (classification unreasonable); *Metropolitan Casualty Ins. Co. vs. Brownell;* 294 U. S. 580, 1935 (classification reasonable).
43. Sickle cell testing statutes include GA. CODE ANN. §88-1201.1 (1973) (newborns); III. Pub. Act 77-2101 (1972) (school children); Ky. Acts ch. 122 (1972) (newborns & marriage applicants); LA. REV. STAT. §17-194 (1973) (School children) and §40-1299.1 (1973) (newborns); Mass. Acts & Resolves ch. 491 (1971) (school children); Miss. Gen. Laws ch. 414 (1972) (school children);

N. Y. DOMESTIC REL. LAW § 13-aa (McKinney 1973) (marriage applicants) & N. Y. ED. LAW § 903 (McKinney 1973) (school children); Va. Acts ch. 778 (1972) (school children); cf. ARIZ. REV. STAT. ANN. § § 36-797.41 & -797.42 (1973) (school children by consent of parent).

A new Domestic Relations Act proposed by the Chicago Bar Association in 1973 contains the provision (§ 206(d)) that a marriage license may only be issued upon presentation to the county clerk of a certificate signed by a licensed physician "setting forth that such person . . . is free from veneral disease, and has been advised of abnormalities which may cause birth defects, as nearly as can be determined by a thorough physical examination and such standard laboratory tests as are necessary for discovery of such diseases."

44. *McCulloch vs. Maryland,* 4 Wheat. 316 (1819).
45. *New York vs. O'Neill,* 359 U. S. 1, 6 (1959).
46. *West Coast Hotel Co. vs. Parrish,* 300 U. S. 379 (1937).
47. *Meyer vs. Nebraska,* 262 U. S. 390 (1923). The "due process" clause of the Fifth Amendment is binding on the federal government while the same clause in the Fourteenth Amendment controls state action.
48. 198 U. S. 45 (1905).
49. Id. at 56.
50. Id. at 58.
51. *United States vs. Carolene Products Co.,* 304 U. S. 104 (1938). See also note 53 infra.
52. We shall discuss only the United States Constitution although many states have provisions in their constitutions which duplicate or resemble the federal requirements of due process and equal protection. To the extent that these state provisions track the national ones, they would probably impose the same restrictions on state genetic programs, and to the extent that the state provisions differ from the national there would be too many variations to discuss here.
53. The groundwork for this distinction was laid by Justice Stone in his famous fourth footnote in *United States vs. Carolene Products Co.,* 304 U. S. 144, 152 (1938). To the holding in the test that "legislation affecting ordinary commercial transactions" was not to be invalidated unless it was completely lacking in rational basis, he added a note that: "There may be narrower scope for operation of the presumption of constitutionality when legislation appears on its face to be within a specific prohibition of the Constitution, such as those of the first ten amendments . . ." Similar reasoning has also applied to "fundamental rights" not explicitly mentioned in the Bill of Rights. See text accompanying note 59 infra; see also *Griswold vs. Connecticut,* 381 U. S. 479, 482 (1965).
54. Although the equal protection clause of the Fourteenth Amendment is applicable by its terms only to state governmental action, its requirement of nondiscrimination has been extended to actions of the federal government under the Fifth Amendment. *Bolling vs. Sharpe,* 347 U. S. 497 (1954).
55. See eg, *Sherbert vs. Verner,* 374 U. S. 398 (1963) (religion); *NAACP vs. Button,* 371 U. S. 415 (1963) (speech). In some cases, explicit and implicit rights, plus the guarantee of equal protection of the laws, are mixed in together. See, for example, the cases dealing with the right to an equal, effective vote, *Dunn vs. Blumstein,* 405 U. S. 331 (1972); *Williams vs. Rhodes,* 393 U. S. 23 (1968); *Harper vs. Virginia Bd. of Elections,* 383 U. S. 663 (1966); *Reynolds vs. Sims,* 377 U. S. 533 (1964).

56. See eg, *Stanley vs. Georgia,* 394 U. S. 557 (1969); *Griswold vs. Connecticut,* 381 U. S. 479 (1965).
57. *Roe vs. Wade,* 410 U. S. 113 (1973).
58. *Snyder vs. Massachusetts,* 291 U. S. 97, 105 (1934).
59. In most cases, legislative classifications of persons into groups, like other types of legislation involving regulations and restrictions, need only be rationally related to a legitimate state interest and not discriminate invidiously, as on the basis of race. See notes 38-42 and accompanying text, supra. But classifications which deny certain persons or groups their fundamental rights "must be closely scrutinized and carefully confined." *Harper vs. Virginia Bd. of Elections,* 383 U. S. 663, 670 (1966). See also notes 91-96 and accompanying text, infra.
60. Eg, *Stanley vs. Georgia,* 394 U. S. 557 (1969) (mere private possession of obscene materials may not be made a crime); *Griswold vs. Connecticut,* 381 U. S. 479 (1965) (statute penalizing possession or use of contraceptives invalid).
61. See eg, *Pierce vs. Society of Sisters,* 268 U. S. 510 (1925); *Meyer vs. Nebraska,* 262 U. S. 390 (1923). See also *Maynard vs. Hill,* 125 U. S. 190 (1888).
62. *Loving vs. Virginia,* 388 U. S. 1, 12 (1967).
63. *Skinner vs. Oklahoma,* 316 U. S. 535, 541 (1942).
64. *Eisenstadt vs. Baird,* 405 U. S. 438 (1972); *Griswold vs. Connecticut,* 381 U. S. 479 (1965).
65. 381 U. S. 479 (1965).
66. Id. at 486.
67. In a concurring opinion Justice Goldberg, joined by the Chief Justice and Justice Brennan, concluded that "the concept of liberty . . . embraces the right of marital privacy though that right is not mentioned explicitly in the Constitution." Id. at 486. He found constitutional support for his position in the Ninth Amendment which "shows a belief of the Constitution's authors that fundamental rights exist that are not expressly enumerated in the first eight amendments." Id. at 492.
68. Id. at 485.
69. 405 U. S. 438 (1972).
70. Id. at 453 (emphasis in original).
71. 410 U. S. 112 (1973).
72. Id. at 153.
73. Id. at 162-63.
74. Id. at 163.
75. Id. at 165.
76. The genetic rationale for prohibiting consanguineous marriages is to reduce the probability that the marriage partners will both carry the same recessive deleterious gene, inherited from a common ancestor. The problem with the laws from a genetics viewpoint is that some prohibit one mating (eg, aunt-nephew) but not another (eg, uncle-niece) of like consanguinity, and that a larger number prohibit affinous as well as consanguineous marriages (ie, prohibit marrying an uncle, whether he is either parent's brother or brother-in-law).
77. *Olmstead vs. United States,* 277 U. S. 438, 478 (1928) (Brandeis, J., dissenting).
78. 410 U. S. at 154.
79. 197 U. S. 11 (1905).
80. Id. at 36.
81. Id.

82. Id. at 29.
83. See *Peterson vs. Widule,* 157 Wis. 641, 147 N. W. 966 (1914).
84. 274 U. S. 200 (1927).
85. Id. at 207.
86. 316 U. S. 535 (1942). Skinner was ordered sterilized under a statute permitting sterilization of "habitual criminals" convicted at least twice for crimes "amounting to felonies involving moral turpitude." The legislation applied to robbers, such as Skinner (who had stolen chickens), but exempted embezzlers, among others. Applying the "strict scrutiny" due a law which infringed a fundamental right, the Supreme Court held that the statute violated the equal protection clause because it drew a distinction between classes of criminals which was unrelated to the purposes of the law.
87. Id. at 541.
88. 274 U. S. at 206.
89. As previously pointed out, however, the physical intrusion involved in mandatory screening is much less than that involved in sterilization, which may reduce the need for justification.
90. See eg, *Argersinger vs. Hamlin*, 407 U. S. 25 (1972); *Shapiro vs. Thompson,* 394 U. S. 618 (1969).
91. *Williamson vs. Lee Optical Co.,* 348 U. S. 483, 489 (1955).
92. *Railway Express vs. New York,* 336 U. S. 106 (1949).
93. 379 U. S. 184 (1964).
94. Id. at 196.
95. 388 U. S. 1 (1967).
96. For example, the stringency of the judge's review might turn on whether there were criminal penalties for noncompliance. See *Loving vs. Virginia,* 388 U. S. 1, 11 (1967); *Korematsu vs. United States,* 323 U. S. 214, 216 (1944).

Mass Screening and Genetic Counseling in Mendelian Disorders

Richard W. Erbe, M.D.

Consideration of the existing mass screening programs for mendelian or single-gene diseases and carrier states makes readily apparent the heterogeneity of the rationales on which they are based. Many of the mass screening programs for inborn errors of metabolism were begun almost as soon as a technically satisfactory method for their detection became available, while most had the additional goals of case finding for epidemiologic and other research purposes, and therapy of affected individuals thus identified. In contrast to programs intended to screen primarily for affected individuals, the most extensive carrier state screening and genetic counseling programs to date are those for sickle cell trait and the Tay-Sachs carrier state.

The purposes of this discussion are to examine the possibilities for additional mass screening and genetic counseling programs for mendelian carrier states and disorders, and to pose at least some of the questions raised by these possible programs. In the discussion it is assumed that future decisions regarding which programs are actually begun, and when, will result from consideration of the following factors: (1) the frequency of the carrier state disease, (2) the burden imposed on physical and psychologic health by the disease, (3) the degree to which the screening and counseling program is perceived as offering a helpful alternative to those at risk, (4) the availability of accurate, relatively simple and inexpensive methods for identifying the carrier state or disease, and (5) the availability of adequate genetic counseling as an integral part of the program. While ideally these factors may ultimately be evaluated in more precise, quantitative terms, the present state of knowledge in medical genetics forces us to rely heavily on subjective judgments. (See the papers

---

Richard W. Erbe, M.D., *Assistant Professor of Pediatrics, Harvard Medical School, Genetics Unit, Massachusetts General Hospital, Boston.*

in this series by Powledge and by Lappé and Roblin for an elaboration of this view.)

More than 1,800 mendelian or single-gene disorders have been described,[1] but the frequencies of many of these entities are unknown. Although the argument can be considered somewhat circular, our knowledge of the frequencies and burdens of many genetic diseases is incomplete as a result of the fact that population surveys of sufficient scope and duration have never been carried out. In many instances such studies have been considered unrewarding when done for purely epidemiologic reasons. Yet the possibility that the frequency of a given carrier state or disease might ultimately prove to be low has been used to negate certain proposed mass screening and counseling programs which would generate valid epidemiologic data in addition to serving other goals, such as counseling and treatment. However, since many of these disorders appear to be exceedingly rare, the overall incidence is determined predominantly by those few disorders of greatest frequency. It can thus be estimated that serious mendelian diseases affect a total of over 1%, or at the most about 2%, of the general population. For analysis, this group of disorders must be further subdivided according to mode of inheritance.

Autosomal Dominant Disorders

More than 940 autosomal dominants have been described.[1] The most common serious disorder or related group of disorders involves elevated plasma lipids, which may affect 1% of the general population,[2,3] and is associated with premature vascular disease. Since the Genetics Group of the Institute first considered the prospects of mass screening and counseling in September 1971, new information has made hyperlipidemia an even more interesting subject for analysis, and so the considerations involved will be reviewed in some detail.

Nearly half the U.S. population dies of arteriosclerosis most often involving the cardiac and less often the cerebral and renal vessels. The best indicator to date that coronary artery disease will occur is an increased concentration of certain plasma lipids.[4] It has been shown that about 5% of adults have an elevated blood cholesterol, and another 5% (only partially overlapping), an increase in triglycerides. Thus, about 7% of the total population, irrespective of race and ethnic origin, seem to have readily identifiable hyperlipidemia by these criteria. In a given individual, when hyperlipidemia is detected, a variety of diseases (eg liver disease, thyroid disease, blood protein abnormalities, etc.) and environmental factors (eg abnormal fat intake, alcoholism, use of certain oral contraceptives, etc.) must be identified when present. Often both of these groups of etiologies are eliminated and family studies disclose similar lipid abnormalities in relatives. It is this latter group, those with *primary familial hyperlipidemia,* with which we are presently concerned. While a large number of investigators have contributed significantly to knowledge of these disorders, the classification of these disorders proposed by Fredrickson et al has been particularly useful.[5,6] According to this schema, these families and individuals can be classified into five identifiable but somewhat overlapping groups by chemical (AutoAnalyzer) and physical (plasma electrophoresis and ultracentrifugation) analysis of the distribution and quantity of their plasma lipoproteins. Of the five types, type II is of particular interest because of its frequent occurrence, its autosomal dominant mode of transmission and the predisposition to premature arteriosclerosis which it produces, a predisposition shared by types III and IV.[6]

According to the studies of Fredrickson and Levy, type II, or *familial hyperbetalipoproteinemia,* is the commonest and most extensively characterized of the hyperlipoproteinemias.[6] There appear to be no racial or ethnic barriers to its occurrence. Single-gene, autosomal dominant transmission appears now to be firmly established.[7] As might be expected where the gene for an autosomal dominant disorder is common, both heterozygotes and homozygotes have been observed. In the less common homozygote, the blood lipid abnormalities are more extreme, xanthomas appear before the age of 10 years and vascular disease usually is manifest before the age of 20. Diagnostic criteria for the homozygote include demonstration of the type II abnormality in both parents.

By contrast, the heterozygote has less extreme (one half to one third of the homozygous levels) but no less characteristic abnormalities of blood lipids, less extensive and later appearing xanthomas and vascular disease, and evidence of type II disease in one or more first-degree relatives. Twenty or more years are required before coronary artery disease begins to appear among the heterozygotes. Recent studies of 104 heterozygotes showed the mean age of onset of coronary artery disease was 43 years in men and 53 years in women. For men the chance of a first heart attack was 5% by age 30, 51% by age 50 and 85% by age 60. For women, the risks were 0 by age 30, 12% by age 50 and 58% by age 60.[8,9] Studies of families ascertained for various reasons suggest the disorder breeds true, in contrast to the less extensive data on the other types. The gene is thought to be completely penetrant. The exclusion of phenocopies is particularly important.[10] Phenocopies can be produced in individuals and families by a diet unusually high in cholesterol and saturated fats. Further, other inherited diseases, including porphyria and familial hypothyroidism, can produce identical patterns of elevated lipids in addition to their own characteristic manifestations.

Therapy by modification of the fat composition of the diet and the addition of one or more drugs is often relatively successful in lowering the blood lipids and even producing resolution of the skin lesions in the heterozygotes. Unfortunately, however, at present there are not sufficient data to decide whether treatment will prevent the development of the vascular complications or, for that matter, even that the treatments proposed are themselves free of toxic effects.[11] It has been argued that treatment should optimally begin in childhood in order to demonstrate a protective effect.[12,13] Treatment of homozygotes results in a considerably more varied and less dramatic response.

Glueck et al[2] surveyed umbilical-cord blood cholesterol levels in 1,800 consecutive unselected live births in a general hospital with more extensive follow-up lipid analysis and family studies. Fourteen infants were identified as having type II disease by the presence of the characteristic plasma lipid abnormalities and the identification of one affected parent with type II disease. These figures, along with the probability that additional type II disease was present in some infants whose parents could not be studied, suggest a frequency of about 1% of the general population and demonstrate the feasibility of conducting such studies in newborns with clear implications regarding a possible prospective study of the effects of therapy from birth.[2,12,14-16]

Other modes of ascertainment of hyperlipidemic patients have given different results with regard to the classification and distribution of the dominantly inherited hyperlipidemias. Recently Goldstein et al[3] carried out extensive studies of 500 survivors of myocardial infarction and found that 31% had hyperlipidemia. Family studies showed that three apparently distinct autosomal dominant disorders accounted for 20% of survivors below 60 years of age. While differing with some previous studies in regard to the relative frequencies of the hyperlipidemias, these authors also arrived at an estimated heterozygote frequency in the general population of about 1%. It may be relevant to note here that about half of the deaths from coronary artery disease occur suddenly and outside the hospital,[17] raising the possibility of ascertainment bias when patients who survive long enough to reach the hospital are studied.

To date most studies of the hyperlipoproteinemias have focused on the relationship between plasma lipid abnormalities and premature vascular disease. Where treatment is involved there are many apparent problems. Diagnosis at birth seems to be a strong present possibility. There is no clearly "best" therapeutic regimen. The alternative therapies involve extensive manipulation of the diet and perhaps also of physical activity levels. One or more expensive drugs might be used and each has its spectrum of side-effects. Therapy would be required throughout two or more decades between diagnosis at birth and the expected onset of cardiovascular disease. During that interval it seems unlikely that the observed results, unless particularly striking, would be a sufficient basis on which to modify the therapy assigned at the time of diagnosis. There would seem to be enormous potential for stigmatization of a heterozygote thus identified both in terms of self-image and in relation to insurers, employers, etc.

Yet the genetic implications are equally staggering. How should we deal with genes of this frequency? Most of our experiences to date with mass screening and counseling involve diseases which are substantially less common even among the particular groups in which they are most likely to occur. Are there as yet unidentified, positive selective factors to account for the fact that the gene frequency is so high? Even though the morbidity and mortality in these disorders occur predominantly in the postreproductive years, some mechanism for maintaining the high gene frequencies seems necessary and positive selection is one possibility (although other mechanisms, such as close linkage to genes under strong positive selection and extraordinarily high mutation rate at these loci, are by no means ruled out). With a high recurrence risk and risk of transmission, as well as at least a moderately serious potential burden, what genetic counseling should be transmitted to screenees; and would this affect their reproductive behavior in view of the fact that the gene is so common? Since so many matings would be considered at high risk for hyperlipoproteinemia, would the total impact of mass genetic counseling be perceived as helpful or harmful? Which of the reproductive alternatives could be meaningfully utilized here? Perhaps prenatal diagnosis will become possible through fetal blood sampling once this technic is perfected, or indirectly by linkage analysis or possibly even the detection of a lipid defect in amniotic fluid cells. If so and if parents wished not to give birth to affected children, should we or could we respond to requests to abort as many as 1 in 200 pregnancies for this disorder alone?

It would be inappropriate to even attempt to answer these questions in view of the present lack of relevant information, but several assertions and speculations may be in order. Faced with overwhelming evidence of a readily identifiable genetic component in the etiology of premature vascular disease, geneticists should involve themselves in new or ongoing studies of hyperlipidemia in order to help insure that genetically valid and relevant data are collected. One might predict a greater parental interest in and acceptance of genetic information regarding a predisposition to coronary artery disease since the public awareness of the disease and its consequences is so great. Since it may require many years before the effectiveness and safety of diet and therapies can be established, a high priority should be placed on the development of technics for the diagnosis of these disorders in utero; once this is achieved, consideration should be given to offering pilot genetic counseling programs with provision for careful assessment of their impact. It thus appears appropriate and timely for geneticists to involve themselves in this common and important group of inherited disorders.

Turning from the inherited hyperlipidemias, let us consider the remaining autosomal dominant disorders. Although many additional serious autosomal dominant diseases have been described, nearly all are unlikely candidates for mass screening and genetic counseling purposes in the foreseeable future, primarily because they are much less common and often no method of screening the general population exists. A possible exception is *multiple neurofibromatosis* regarding which extensive data are available from the classic study of Crow, Schull and Neel.[18] The incidence of this disorder in Michigan was estimated at 1/2,500 to 3,300, making this perhaps the second most frequent serious autosomal dominant disorder. Nearly 80% of persons with neurofibromatosis had six or more cafe-au-lait spots of significant size, while no normals were found to have this degree of abnormal cutaneous pigmentation. One could consider the possibility of mass screening by using the cafe-au-lait spots to identify persons suspected of having neurofibromatosis, since these persons are otherwise less likely to be aware of the presence of this gene. This approach, however, would have serious drawbacks in that several diseases other than neurofibromatosis can produce cafe-au-lait spots, and not all the persons with the gene for neurofibromatosis develop the skin lesions or other serious complications, thus introducing the possibility of significant errors in genetic counseling. Furthermore, prenatal diagnosis is not possible in neurofibromatosis, restricting the reproductive usefulness of the information thus gained, and there is nearly nothing in the way of therapy which could delay or prevent the more serious manifestations of the disease. Thus there appears to be little basis for suggesting mass screening and counseling for multiple neurofibromatosis.

Familial adenomatosis colonic polyposis, or gastrointestinal polyposis type I, is another autosomal dominant disorder and occurs with an estimated frequency of 1/8,300.[19] Its inheritance is clearly established, and the gene is probably completely penetrant although the expressivity in terms of the number of colonic polyps is variable. Of paramount importance, 70% or more of individuals with this disease will develop carcinoma of the colon by the age of 40 years if the disease is not treated by colectomy.[20] With the potential for great benefit to individuals affected with this disease which occurs more frequently than, for example, phenylketonuria, mass screening might be considered. Again, however, there are drawbacks. The multiple colonic polyps can develop in the first decade or not until later. Mass screening would require extensive and repeated bowel examinations and thus is a practical impossibility. Prenatal diagnosis is presently impossible in this disorder as well as in the over 900 other autosomal dominant disorders, except for one. In the rare disease *myotonic dystrophy,* intrauterine diagnosis is possible by taking advantage of the close linkage between the locus for myotonic dystrophy and that for ABH-secretor, the latter being detectable in amniotic fluid.[21]

Similar analyses in terms of the five factors outlined in the introduction of other autosomal dominants indicate that mass screening and counseling is not a useful approach. Rather, it seems appropriate at present to continue the traditional practice of close examination and genetic counseling of the relatives of affected individuals.

Autosomal Recessive Disorders

Nearly 800 autosomal recessive disorders have been described.[1] These will be considered only briefly in this section. Two of the most common, sickle cell anemia and Tay-Sachs disease and their carrier states, are the foci for much of the discussion in this volume. Cystic fibrosis has received considerable attention but at present there exists no generally accepted method for mass carrier state screening. Since, as is well known, cystic fibrosis occurs almost exclusively in Caucasians, the development of carrier state screening capability would have the ancillary benefit of broadening the racial orientation of mass screening and genetic counseling programs.

A group of autosomal recessive disorders for which mass screening has recently been begun involve serum alpha$_1$-antitrypsin and the protease inhibitor (Pi) alleles.[22] More than 20 alleles have been distinguished and, when appropriate physical and activity measurements are used in combination,[23] certain Pi genotypes have been found to be associated with disease. Individuals with the severe $alpha_1$-antitrypsin deficiency state have the Pi type ZZ and 10%-15% of normal trypsin inhibitory capacity in serum. It appears that about 10% of Pi ZZ individuals die of juvenile cirrhosis, while some 80% develop pulmonary emphysema in early adulthood.[24] In Sweden, a total of 23,800 infants have been screened for $alpha_1$-antitrypsin deficiency using capillary blood obtained on the fourth to sixth day following birth, and spotted and dried on filter paper for semiquantitative immunoassay.[24] The data thus obtained were compared with those found by slightly different methods in adults screened in both Oslo and St. Louis. The results show an incidence of Pi ZZ in newborns of 1/1,041, the frequency of the Z carrier state thus being 1/17. In contrast, adults in St. Louis showed a Pi ZZ frequency of 1/5,917 and a Z carrier state frequency of 1/40, while the corresponding frequencies in Oslo were 1/3,906 for Pi ZZ and 1/32 for the Z carrier state.[24] Longitudinal studies are planned to determine whether the decreased frequencies of Pi ZZ in adults are due to mortality related to the $alpha_1$-antitrypsin, to differences in the analytic methods used or to factors as yet unidentified.

In contrast to the severe deficiency seen in Pi ZZ, intermediate deficiencies occur with the Pi genotypes MZ and SS.[23] Particularly timely questions have been raised as to whether such individuals may be predisposed to chronic pulmonary diseases and whether they should be advised to avoid occupational or other exposure to fumes, dust, smoke, etc. which might accelerate the rate of pathologic lung changes.[25]

It would appear that it is now not only technically feasible but of great potential value to carry out mass screening studies of $alpha_1$-antitrypsin deficiency. Much additional information needs to be gained regarding the medical burden of various Pi genotypes, especially ZZ, SS and MZ, through longitudinal studies before accurate genetic counseling is possible. Such longitudinal studies have been under way for a relatively short time, and the results of many previous studies of liver disease in childhood and premature lung disease in adults are limited by ascertainment bias since the $alpha_1$-antitrypsin testing was directed at those already having hepatic or lung disease. At present no specific treatment of $alpha_1$-antitrypsin deficiency is known. Although easily measured in serum, $alpha_1$-antitrypsin has not been detected to date in extracts of cultured amniotic fluid cells. Perhaps prenatal diagnosis will become possible here, too, when methods for obtaining blood from the 14- to 16-week fetus have been devised. When all of these factors are considered it appears that there is potentially much to be gained both medically and genetically through further assessment of these relatively common, autosomal recessively inherited $alpha_1$-antitrypsin deficiency states. As a result of such studies it may in the relatively near future be possible to add these disorders to those already being sought in mass screening and genetic counseling programs (See the paper by Lappé and Roblin in this series.)

X-Linked Recessive Disorders

Fully 150 X-linked recessive disorders have been described.[1] Certainly the most common in the United States, as well as worldwide, is *glucose-6-phosphate dehydrogenase* (G-6-PD) *deficiency.*[26] In the United States, the predominant deficiency is associated with the variant designated A^- which affects approximately 11%-12% of black males. Exposure to certain oxidant drugs, such as antimalarials, produces hemolysis is these individuals, but it is usually mild and not a serious threat to health. Because of its general course and since this hemolysis is preventable by avoiding the drugs which promote hemolysis, the burden of this disorder is generally perceived as mild. The major reason for mass screening, where this is done, has been to detect the G-6-PD deficient males in order to advise them to avoid the provocative drugs, rather than for genetic counseling.

Other X-linked recessive disorders occur at considerably lower frequency, although some, such as *Duchenne muscular dystrophy,* impose a heavy burden and are widely recognized as serious by the general public.

Consideration of the factors outlined in the introduction raises the possibility that we should now take steps to initiate mass screening and genetic counseling programs to screen for the carrier state of *hemophilia A* or X-linked hemophilia. Knowledge of this disease dates to antiquity with the Talmudic fatal exsanguination following circumcision of the sons of several sisters. More recently, it seems likely that Queen Victoria was a carrier of hemophilia A, since two of her granddaughters gave birth to sons with hemophilia – one of whom was Alexis Tsarevich, the only son and heir of Nicholas II, the last Tsar of Russia.[27] The X-linked pattern was described in 1803 and the coagulation defect in 1893; since that time there has been steady progress in understanding the pathophysiologies of this and related disorders of hemostasis.[28] During this time it has become apparent that there are a number of separate disorders grouped under the general heading of hemophilia and that these are inherited in different mendelian patterns.[29] Precise diagnosis in any given family has relied heavily on laboratory technics which have not always provided a clear distinction between these genetically heterogeneous entities.

Hemophilia A, however, is generally the most serious of these and has received considerable attention. That this disease imposes a heavy physical, emotional and financial burden on affected males and their families is well documented. For example, Meyers et al[30] studied in detail 70 hemophilic patients and their families, supplementing the medical records with interviews and questionnaires. Of the 70 patients, 20 had severe hemophilia with a factor VIII activity of less than 1% of normal, while 7 had moderate (1%-5% of normal) and 43 mild (5%-30% of normal) factor VIII deficiency. A number of patients had received less than optimal medical care as judged by other physicians and the patients themselves. Marked family stresses were apparent. The patients often perceived themselves, and were viewed by parents, as a burden to the activities and resources of the family and a source of nervous tension. While there was a general correlation of these perceptions with the severity of the disease, nonetheless, even the mild hemophilics with infrequent bleeding episodes were the source of considerable tension. While the families of mild hemophiliacs showed an inverse correlation between expressed fear and understanding of the disease, no such beneficial effect was apparent in the families of moderate and severe hemophiliacs. There were recurrent conflicts between parents and sons regarding sports and other vigorous activities, the parents encouraging the substitution of intellectual achievement. Problems in schooling were expressed and, in adults, major problems in employment, including difficulties in obtaining a job, loss of time from work, placement in inappropriate jobs (eg as a meat cutter). About half of the hemophiliacs and parents saw the disease as a reason for limiting family size, but, of these, 35% lacked the information needed for family planning.

Much additional information has been provided as part of the National Heart and Lung Institute's Blood Resource Studies report.[31] A broad range of major treatment centers, physicians, patients and their families were surveyed. Results disclosed that during 1970 and 1971 some 25,500 persons in the United States were treated for severe or moderate hemophilia. Although no direct psychosocial assessment was attempted in this survey, a considerable burden was evident. Hemophilia interfered with educational opportunities, with 65% of those under age 16 reporting poor school attendance. Of those over age 16, 40% were unemployed and half gave poor health as the primary reason. About 60% of the families spent an average of $2,000 per year on blood products and other related care, while maximum costs ran as high as $65,000. Although hemophiliacs are unable to purchase major medical insurance, many received coverage as part of family health insurance policies or public and private sources, and only 3% reported that they were unable to obtain needed care. In order to meet the costs not covered by insurance, 20% of fathers found it necessary to work one or more extra jobs and one third of the mothers took jobs for reasons attributed directly to the costs of hemophilia treatment. In over half of the 25,500 patients, serious bleeding necessitated some form of treatment by the age of 1 year and the intravenous infusion of blood products before the age of 6. Some 95% of the treatment was given in response to frank bleeding episodes, while only 5% was given on a prophylactic basis with periodic administration generally three times per week to prevent bleeding episodes. The treatment of these patients with severe factor VIII deficiency required the equivalent of 2.3 million units of whole blood out of the approximately 9.3 million units of whole blood and 1.7 million units of plasma collected during 1971. Thus the treatment of hemophilia A consumes a substantial portion of the blood and blood products in the United States. If prophylactic therapy, which has been advocated by some,[32-34] were adopted, the treatment of severe factor VIII deficient patients would require the equivalent of some 13 million units of blood annually. In the face of current shortages of blood, the problems in blood banks and the federal policy requiring blood banks to shift from largely paid to entirely unpaid donors, questions have been raised here and elsewhere[35] about how this large medical burden is to be supported.

Recent advances in immunochemical assay methods for detecting factor VIII[36-38] have made it possible to distinguish hemophilia A from the other hemophilia syndromes.[29] Hemophilia A is characterized by a marked reduction of plasma factor VIII activity, but normal plasma levels of immunoreactive factor VIII protein. When the functional (clot-promoting) factor VIII assay is used in combination with a quantitative immunoelectrophoretic assay, it has been shown to be possible to detect female carriers in families already having at least one hemophilic male[39] with far greater accuracy than previously, when the functional factor VIII assay alone was used. With accurate tests for the carrier state now available, mass screening of women to detect carriers and provide genetic counseling *prior* to the birth of the first affected son should be considered.

Data regarding reproduction and even life expectancy of persons with severe hemophilia A are lacking. It is possible with some assumptions, however, to estimate the potential impact of such a screening and counseling program. From the data in the NHLI report,[31] the estimated prevalence of severe factor VIII deficiency is 1/8,600 males with a median patient population age of 11.5 years. In view of the mortality rate of this disease the incidence at birth is probably even higher, although lower incidence figures have been reported.[30,40] However, using the frequency of 1/8,600 males, it is possible to estimate the frequency of prereproductive women who carry the gene for severe hemophilia A but have no affected males in the present generation (ie brothers or cousins) or preceding generation (ie uncles) to otherwise identify them. Since until recently most severe hemophiliacs have been thought not to reproduce, almost one third of the genes for this disease were lost each generation. It has therefore been assumed that about one third of the genes for hemophilia A have arisen in each generation by new mutations, of which two thirds occur in females. Thus a female can become a carrier of hemophilia A either by inheriting a gene from her mother or through the process of fresh mutation. Assuming that the average family has three children, it can be calculated that about 1 prereproductive female in every 10,000 is a carrier of severe hemophilia A and has no affected brother, cousin or uncle. Regardless of whom she marries, each such carrier runs a 50% risk of hemophilia in each son, and each of her daughters has a 50% risk of inheriting the carrier state.

At present, for hemophilia carriers thus identified, one reproductive alternative consists of prenatal sex determination with abortion of male fetuses. While hemophilia A occurs among all ethnic and racial groups, an accurate prenatal diagnosis of affected males can now be made if the carrier mother has inherited the gene from a previous generation in about 50% of black hemophilia carriers,[41] by taking advantage of the close linkage of the hemophilia A and glucose-6-phosphate dehydrogenase loci.[42,43] Whether prenatal diagnosis will become possible in all carriers once technics for obtaining fetal blood are perfected is a matter of conjecture.

The effects of such a mass carrier state screening and genetic counseling program on the incidence of the disease and the frequency of the carrier state obviously depend on the reproductive behavior of carriers thus identified. The possible changes over time have been nicely illustrated by Holloway and Smith.[44] In the extremes, if carrier females have only their intended number of pregnancies after prospective detection, and all males or all affected males are aborted, the frequency of the hemophilia A gene will decrease substantially. If, however, full reproductive compensation occurs (ie the carriers have the intended number of children rather than pregnancies) following prospective detection, and all males are aborted, the gene frequency will actually increase dramatically.

Those who have advocated home treatment programs with self-administration of factor VIII have emphasized the improved health and functioning of the patients thus treated[45-47] in spite of the greater cost of such therapy.[47] As such therapy improves the functioning of these patients, it is a reasonable assumption that the hemophilic males will increasingly father children, because there is no direct effect of this disease on the reproductive system. Since their daughters will be obligate carriers, the contribution of this source of genes for severe hemophilia A must also be considered. In the absence of published data on the fertility of male hemophiliacs, however, it can hardly be considered in quantitative terms.

Finally, even with maximal utilization of such a prospective mass screening and counseling program, the process of mutation will provide a continuing number of males with hemophilia A.

There are many problems of both an ethical and technical nature which would need consideration before such a program could be initiated. However, hemophilia A brings into focus many of the most difficult value judgments which must be faced in any genetic screening program.

In conclusion, review of the over 1,800 mendelian disorders in man indicates that at present only a relatively small number are suitable for mass screening and genetic counseling programs. For each screenable disorder many problems remain to be solved, but these programs will likely be important prototypes as our technical capabilities increase and as society as a whole becomes more aware of the opportunities for prevention of genetic disease which these programs can offer.

References

1. McKusick, V. A.: *Mendelian Inheritance in Man.* Baltimore:Johns Hopkins Press, 1971.
2. Glueck, C. J., Heckman, F., Schoenfeld, M. et al: Neonatal familial type II hyperlipoproteinemia: Cord blood cholesterol in 1800 births. *Metabolism, 6*:597, 1971.
3. Goldstein, J. L., Hazzard, W. R., Schrott, H. G. et al: Hyperlipidemia in coronary heart disease. I. Lipid levels in 500 survivors of myocardial infarction. II. Genetic analysis of lipid levels in 176 families and delineation of a new inherited disorder, combined hyperlipidemia. III. Evaluation of lipoprotein phenotypes of 156 genetically defined survivors of myocardial infarction. *J. Clin. Invest., 52*:1533, 1544, 1569, 1973.
4. Kannel, W. B., Castelli, W.P., Gordon, T. and McNamara, P. M.: Serum cholesterol, lipoproteins, and the risk of coronary heart disease. *Ann. Intern. Med., 74*:1, 1971.
5. Fredrickson, D. S. and Lees, R. S.: A system for phenotyping hyperlipoproteinemia. *Circulation, 31*:321, 1965.

6. Fredrickson, D. S. and Levy, R. I.: Familial hyperlipoproteinemia. In Stanbury, J. B., Wyngaarden, J. B. and Fredrickson, D. S. (eds.): *The Metabolic Basis of Inherited Disease.* New York:McGraw-Hill Book Co., 1972, p. 545.
7. McKusick, V. A.: *Mendelian Inheritance in Man.* Baltimore:Johns Hopkins Press, 1971, p. 159.
8. Slack, J. and Nevin, N. C.: Hyperlipidemic xanthomatosis. I: Increased risk of death from ischaemic heart disease in first degree relatives of 53 patients with essential hyperlipidaemia and xanthomatosis. *J. Med. Genet., 5*:4, 1969.
9. Slack, J.: Risks of ischaemic heart disease in familial hyperlipoproteinemic states. *Lancet, 2*:1380, 1969.
10. Levy, R. I.: Classification and etiology of hyperlipoproteinemias. *Fed. Proc., 30*:829, 1971.
11. *Arteriosclerosis,* report by Task Force on Arteriosclerosis, National Heart and Lung Institute, June, 1971.
12. Glueck, C. J. and Tsang, R. C.: Pediatric familial type II hyperlipoproteinemia: Effects of diet on plasma cholesterol in the first year of life. *Amer. J. Clin. Nutr., 25*:224, 1972.
13. Kannel, W. B. and Dawber, T. R.: Atherosclerosis as a pediatric problem. *J. Pediat., 80*:544, 1972.
14. Kwiterovich, P. O., Jr., Levy, R. I. and Fredrickson, D. S.: Neonatal diagnosis of familial type-II hyperlipoproteinemia. *Lancet, 1*:118, 1973.
15. Blumenthal, S. and Jesse, M. J.: Prevention of atherosclerosis: A pediatric problem. *Hosp. Prac., 4*:81, 1970.
16. Levy, R. I. and Rifkind, B. M.: Diagnosis and management of hyperlipoproteinemia in infants and children. *Amer. J. Cardiol., 31*:547, 1973.
17. Gordon, T. and Kannel, W. B.: Premature mortality from coronary heart disease, the Framingham study. *JAMA, 215*:1617, 1971.
18. Crowe, F. W., Schull, W. J. and Neel, J. V.: *Multiple Neurofibromatosis.* Springfield:Charles C Thomas, 1956.
19. Reed, T. E. and Neel, J. V.: A genetic study of multiple polyposis of the colon (with an appendix deriving a method for estimating relative fitness). *Amer. J. Hum. Genet., 7*:236, 1955.
20. Dukes, C. E.: Pre-cancerous condition of the colon and rectum. *J. Roy. Coll. Surg. Edinb., 3*:182, 1958.
21. Harper, P. S., Rivas, M. L., Bias, W. B. et al: Genetic linkage confirmed between the locus for myotonic dystrophy and the ABH-secretion and Lutheran blood group. *Amer. J. Hum. Genet., 24*:310, 1972.
22. Fagerhol, M. K. and Laurell, C.-B. The *Pi* system-inherited variants of serum α_1-antitrypsin. *Prog. Med. Genet., 7*:96, 1970.
23. Talamo, R. C., Langley, C. E., Levine, B. W. and Kazemi, H.: Genetics vs. quantitative analysis of serum alpha$_1$-antitrypsin. *New Eng. J. Med., 287*:1067, 1973.
24. Laurell, C.-B and Sveger, T.: Mass screening for alpha$_1$-antitrypsin deficiency in newborns. In Mangos, J. A. and Talamo, R. C. (eds.): *Fundamental Problems in Cystic Fibrosis and Related Diseases.* Miami:Symposia Specialists, 1973, p. 269.
25. Lieberman, J.: Alpha$_1$-antitrypsin deficiency. *Med. Clin. N. Amer., 57*:691, 1973.
26. Beutler, E.: Glucose-6-phosphate dehydrogenase deficiency, In Stanbury, J. B., Wyngaarden, J. B. and Frederickson, D. S. (eds.): *The Metabolic Basis of Inherited Disease.* New York:McGraw-Hill Book Co., 1972, p. 1358.

27. Hemophilia. *Medical World News, 12*:64, Nov. 19, 1971.
28. Hougie, C.: Hemophilia and related conditions – Congenital deficiencies of prothrombin (factor II), factor V, and factor VII to XII. In Williams, W. J. et al (eds.): *Hematology*. New York:McGraw-Hill Book Co., 1972, p. 1973.
29. Ratnoff, O. D. and Bennett, B.: The genetics of hereditary disorders of blood coagulation. *Science, 179*:1291, 1973.
30. Meyers, R. D., Adams, W., Dardick, K. et al: The social and economic impact of hemophilia – A survey of 70 cases in Vermont and New Hampshire. *Amer. J. Pub. Health, 62*:530, 1972.
31. *Summary Report: NHLI's Blood Resource Studies,* publication no. (NIH) 73-416. Department of Health, Education and Welfare, Public Health Service, National Institutes of Health, 1972, p. 101.
32. Kasper, C. K., Dietrich, S. L. and Rapaport, S. I.: Hemophilia prophylaxis with factor VIII concentrate. *Arch. Int. Med., 125*:1004, 1970.
33. van Creveld, S.: Prophylaxis of joint hemorrhages in hemophilia. *Acta Haematol., 45*:120, 1971.
34. Lazerson, J.: The prophylactic approach to hemophilia A. *Hosp. Prac., 6*:99, 1971.
35. Treatment of haemophilia, editorial. *Lancet, 2*:648, 1973.
36. Shanberg, J. N. and Gore, I.: Studies on the immunologic and physiologic activities of antihemophilic factor (AHF). *J. Lab. Clin. Med., 50*:954, 1957.
37. Zimmerman, T. S., Ratnoff, O. D. and Powell, A. E.: Immunologic differentiation of classic hemophilia (factor VIII deficiency) and von Willebrand's disease. *J. Clin. Invest., 50*:244, 1971.
38. Hoyer, L. W.: Immunologic studies of antihemophilic factor (AHF, factor VIII). IV. Radioimmunoassay of AHF antigen. *J. Lab. Clin. Med., 80*:822, 1972.
39. Bennett, B. and Ratnoff, O. D.: Detection of the carrier state for classic hemophilia. *New Eng. J. Med., 288*:342, 1973.
40. Stevenson, A. C. and Kerr, C. B.: On the distributions of frequencies of mutations to genes determining harmful traits in man. *Mutat. Res., 4*:339, 1967.
41. Kirkman, H. N.: Linkage and genetic markers in antenatal diagnosis. In Dorfman, A. (ed.): *Antenatal Diagnosis.* Chicago:University of Chicago Press, 1972, p. 57.
42. Boyer, S. H. and Graham, J. B.: Linkage between the X chromosome loci for glucose-6-phosphate dehydrogenase electrophoretic variation and hemophilia A. *Amer. J. Hum. Genet., 17*:320, 1965.
43. McCurdy, P. R.: Use of genetic linkage for the detection of female carriers of hemophilia. *New Eng. J. Med., 285*:218, 1971.
44. Holloway, S. M. and Smith, C.: Equilibrium frequencies in X-linked recessive disease. *Amer. J. Hum. Genet., 25*:388, 1973.
45. Lazerson, J.: Hemophilia home transfusion program: Effect on school attendance. *J. Pediat., 81*:330, 1972.
46. Levin, P. B. and Britten, A. F. H.: Supervised patient-management of hemophilia; A study of 45 patients with hemophilia A and B. *Ann. Int. Med., 78*:195, 1973.
47. Lazerson, J.: Hemophilia home transfusion program: Analysis of cost data. *J. Pediat., 83*:623, 1973.

Screening for Polygenic Disorders

Lee Ehrman, Ph.D. and Marc Lappé, Ph.D.

Introduction

Literally, disease means the "lack of ease." We would like to be able to sharply distinguish as diseases, pathologic states of the body from normal ones. This becomes increasingly difficult, however, when the underlying architecture of the disease in question is genetic and multifactorially so. Multifactorial or *polygenic* (equivalent terms) inheritance almost always precludes a clear segregation into discrete classes, so that good health is likely to blend gradually into what is routinely recognized as a pathologic condition. This shading fosters difficulties in screening, counseling and treatment for such conditions.

In the absence of knowledge concerning specifiable metabolic abnormalities for most if not all *polygenic* disorders (one usually identifies a genetic condition as a "disease" only when its specific etiology is known), screening will often depend on identifying ancillary factors associated with the underlying pathologies. For example, the observation of an increased systolic or diastolic blood pressure may be symptomatic of a hypothetic genetic malresponse to catecholamines, but cannot be said to be diagnostic of this genetic cause. Consequently, as a first stage of screening, agreed-upon indices of some common pathology need to be identified. During this stage, studies of probands and family members will also be done to establish any possible genetic basis for the disorder.

Having established a disease category, the decision to screen for a specific polygenic disorder will then depend on four major criteria: (1) the health burden of the condition, (2) a demonstrable genetic component, (3) available therapeutic modalities, and (4) the existence of suitable tests for presymptomatic detection. Here we will consider only the last three

---

Lee Ehrman, Ph.D., *Associate Professor, Division of Natural Sciences, State University of New York, Purchase and* Marc Lappé, Ph.D., *Associate for the Biological Sciences, Institute of Society, Ethics and Life Sciences, Hastings-on-Hudson, N. Y.*

criteria, since precise determination of the "burden" of any disorder is complex. (See the essay by Gustafson in this series.)

Considering the total burden of human disease, however, it is unquestionable that polygenic disorders occupy a predominant position in contributing to morbidity or mortality or to both. Considering only the genetics of such conditions, screening for diseases of multifactorial hereditary etiology will be the most technically difficult undertaking considered in this survey. Many of the factors which confound the genetic analysis of complex human disease states have been alluded to by Murphy.[1,2]

When familial data, ie conditions recurring in relatives, are inconsistent with autosomal dominant or recessive or X-linked dominant or recessive modes of inheritance, or other relatively simple modes of inheritance (eg neither dominant nor recessive but involving few pairs of genes), one suspects that the data are the result of several genetic loci acting in concert. This action is quantitative and produces a unimodal as distinguished from a bimodal distribution when afflicted plus assorted degrees of partially afflicted and unafflicted subjects in a population are graded[3] (Figs. 1 and 2).

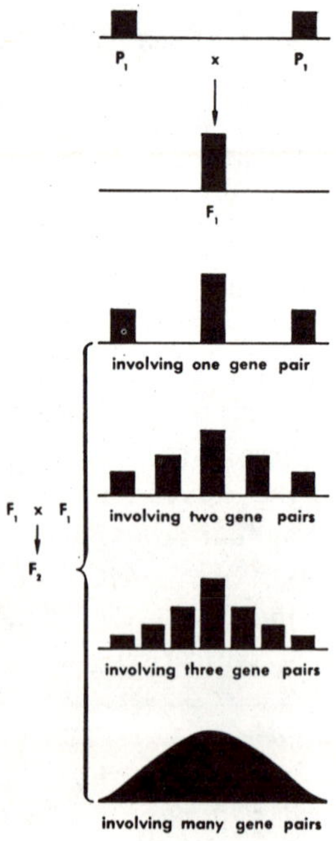

Fig. 1. Distribution of P_1, F_1 and F_2 phenotypes according to the number of segregating pairs of genes. (From Herskowitz.[4])

In part because of this pattern of inheritance, most polygenic conditions are extremely labile with respect to environmental influences and, one would theoretically expect, with regard to therapeutic interventions which potentially might mitigate their expression. It is important to keep the following observations in mind as we turn to specific disorders (refer to Fig. 2):

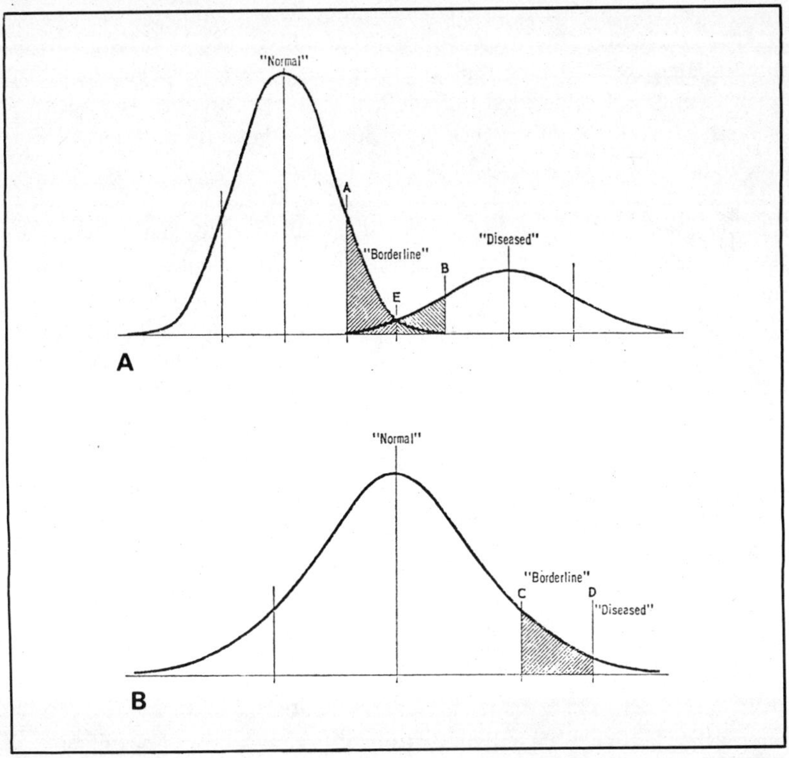

Fig. 2. Distribution of a variable in a population. (A) Bimodal distribution, eg for genetically dominant conditions with incomplete penetrance. (B) Unimodal distribution, eg for polygenic inheritance. This figure illustrates graphically the concepts of sensitivity and specificity. A screening test giving a positive reading at the level of *A* (part A) or *C* (part B) would be highly sensitive, missing few cases but yielding many false-positives; by contrast, the cut-off points at *B* and *D*, respectively, indicate a very specific test. In practice it seems likely that a trial by randomization of treatment should enable a reasonable decision on the cut-off point to be made between those considered in need of treatment and those who may be reassured that they are healthy. (From Wilson and Jungner.[5])

1. "Diseased" and "normal" individuals will often be intergraded.
2. As a result of intergrading, tests for detection which are too sensitive will yield false-positives.
3. Therapeutic interventions need to be titrated against the stage of manifestation of the disorder.
4. Alterations in the environment which may have precipitated disease expression can usually only partially (at best) be later reversed to ameliorate the condition.

In considering putatively polygenic disorders (eg cleft lip, schizophrenia, etc.), we conclude that at present only three – diabetes mellitus, hypertension and the neural tube defects – lend themselves to screening analysis; most of the others have been considered and found wanting. For example, while the development of the fetal amnioscope (discussed below) might permit the in utero detection of a fetus with faulty closure of the maxillary process early in pregnancy, it is unknown to what extent this may simply represent delayed closure or a severe palate deformity. Moreover, no criteria for ranking severity of cleft lip and palate exist which would be applicable in utero. Similar objections exist for neural tube defects, but for these the concordance of a visible anatomic disorder with subsequent disability likely would be good. Schizophrenia, on the other hand, is a highly complex constellation of diagnostic categories with little agreement on its natural course or the long-term efficacy of therapeutic modalities. In contrast, diabetes and hypertension, while complex, follow a predictable course and are amenable to a variety of preemptive therapeutic interventions.

Diabetes Mellitus

Evidence for a Polygenic Etiology

It has been stated that, "Diabetes mellitus is in many respects a geneticist's nightmare. As a disease, it presents almost every impediment to a proper genetic study which can be recognized."[6] In spite of this pessimistic assessment, there is now some general agreement that the bulky and complex data from many sources are often consistent with what is known about multifactorial inheritance. For this reason, screening using glucose tolerance (and cortisone-glucose tolerance) tests may be feasible in adolescents and young adults with family histories of diabetes. Neel et al have shown that in prediabetics or in the diabetically predisposed, there are significant deviations from normal glucose tolerance curves in the 10-29 age interval.[6] On the strength of this and other studies, appropriate tests and medical as well as familial histories provide a mechanism for scoring "definite" or "potential" diabetics, as well as putative "normals." But this is not a disease of sudden onset; so the dividing line between "latent" and "overt" is likely to continue to be obscure.

What may be stated about the genetic aspects of diabetes mellitus? There is little doubt that diabetes shows a familial tendency (Table 1). However, a familial tendency alone is insufficient to establish the genetic nature of diabetes.

For example, it is well to keep in mind that the extreme degree to which environmental factors influence the expression of the diabetic phenotype, plus the variable age of expression of the overt disease combine to confound any simple etiologic analysis. Moreover, as Rimoin has emphasized, "The most important impediment to genetic analysis . . . is the lack of knowledge concerning the basic defect in diabetes."[8]

Because there is no reliable marker for the prediabetic state, both genetic studies and effective prescriptive screening will inevitably be hampered. Ideally we would like to be able to detect all of the individuals who possess a mutant genotype which places them at risk for diabetes; unfortunately, we do not yet have the necessary knowledge to make that determination.

While many often conflicting hypotheses exist for the genetic basis of diabetes,[9-18] there is some agreement that the juvenile form probably has a polygenic basis, with an age-related threshold of expression.[19] However, because diabetes mellitus is manifest phenotypically by an intolerance to glucose whose metabolism is under the control of many different genetic loci, any number of metabolic abnormalities could mimic the diabetic phenotype. Consequently, it is most likely that diabetes represents a heterogeneous condition with multiple possible genetic etiologies.

Table 1. Empiric Risks of Diabetes in First-Degree Relatives of Probands*

Age of Onset of Diabetes in Proband	*% Risk of Occurrence in First-Degree Relatives by Age*			
	25 years	*45 years*	*65 years*	*85 years*
[Population prevalence]	0.18	0.47	1.68	1.37
0-24 yrs old	5-8	5-13	5-17	7-25
25-44 yrs old	1-2	2-4	1-10	12-19
45-64 yrs old	∼1	0.5-3	8-10	13-20
65-84 yrs old	∼1	1-3	6-8	12-22

Note that the risk of occurrence by the age of 25 is substantially higher if a first-degree relative also developed the disease by age 25; this type of evidence suggests, but does not establish, the existence of two distinct kinds of diabetes: early-onset, or juvenile, and late-onset.

*Adapted from Darlow et al.[7]

Therapies

In considering the therapeutic modalities available for treating diabetes, it is well to have in mind the classic sequence of juvenile diabetes. According to Weil,[19] this condition is characterized by

> . . . rapid onset, episodes of hypoglycemia, proneness to ketoacidoses, an almost absolute requirement for insulin and the lack of obesity as an associated finding. The natural history of the illness in children is characterized by four stages. The first, beginning with conception, may be termed prediabetes. The only recognized abnormalities that may exist during this period are in the level of insulin activity and the presence of insulin antagonists in the serum. The second stage, subclinical diabetes, is a period during which stress resulting from illness, surgery, trauma or emotional upheavals will produce a detectable abnormality in carbohydrate metabolism. In this stage carbohydrate metabolism appears to be normal during intervening periods. The second stage may last for several months to many years. The third stage, latent diabetes, is usually brief in children and is defined as a period when the glucose tolerance is abnormal, but fasting blood sugars are within the normal range. The fourth stage is overt diabetes, when insulin treatment is required. At the end of this period the total diabetic state ensues and is present the remainder of the individual's life.

Obviously, different therapeutic modalities will have different effects depending on the stage of the illness. The initial pathologic manifestations are largely confined to the consequences of proliferative changes in blood vessel walls. These include microaneurysms in the retina, some glomerular damage and incipient arteriosclerosis, and may be reversible upon institution of early therapy.[cf 5,20] Commenting on the relative value of therapies instituted in early childhood, Wilson and Jungner note that any therapeutic modality (dietetic or insulin-related) which maintains the urine sugar-free will have beneficial effects on minimizing these sequelae as well as the later appearing cataracts and neuropathies.[5] Basic treatment includes weight reduction, proper diet and exercise or drugs like the biguanides which increase the efficiency of glucose utilization.* In considering all modalities, Wilson and Jungner conclude:

> There is therefore a considerable body of evidence (though open to the objection of selection between groups) in favour of the benefits of treatment in minimizing diabetic complications. It must also be allowed that there is some evidence to the contrary, particularly on the progress of retinopathy and renal changes.[5]

---

*Other insulinotrophic drugs might also be considered, such as sulphonylurea.

Detection

Screening may be directed towards detecting increased urinary (glycosuria) or blood (glycemia) levels of glucose. Urine screening has been widely undertaken, but it is the glucose tolerance test, or the combined glucose-corticosteroid test which apparently affords the best prospect of early detection. Urine screening is frequently unreliable, especially in testing the elderly, since these and other individuals may have high renal thresholds for glucose.[21]

Unfortunately, there is no universal agreement as to what constitutes a positive test. While there is widespread acceptance of the two-hour capillary blood-sugar estimation, there is little agreement as to what constitutes a definitive positive test. For example, WHO recommends a level of 140 mg% value for glucose two hours after testing, while others take 200 mg% as the diagnostic level. (Cited in Wilson and Jungner.[5]) However, there is agreement that it is critically important to keep fasting times constant prior to the test.[22]

The general conclusion about the advisability of diabetes screening depends in part on the objectives of the program. For example, Butterfield believes that prescriptive screening could detect 50% of all unsuspected diabetics, but the desirability of introducing such screening early in life has been seriously questioned for lack of understanding of the results of introducing different therapeutic options.[20] Indeed, it is still the case that in the absence of better knowledge about the etiology of the disease, we are treating the symptoms and not the underlying causes.

Hypertension

Evidence for a Polygenic Etiology

The recent literature is replete with unsupported statements which imply a genetic basis for hypertension. Robinson,[23] for example, states that "since hypertension is inherited, when grouped in families it is usually more serious." While there is ample evidence for *some* genetic factor(s) in hypertension (to be reviewed below), there are many ancillary factors which contribute to (or may be the proximal causative factors in) hypertension. Among the most commonly cited factors in the pathogenesis of hypertension are plasma volume, hormones (eg renin), catecholamines (eg norepinephrine) and enzymes which activate agents with vasoactive capabilities (eg kallikrein and bradykinin). Some of these factors and their putative interrelationships in hypertension are schematically shown in Figure 3.

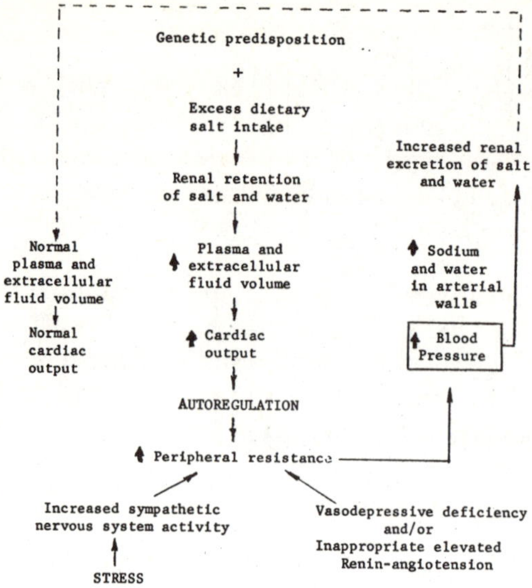

Fig. 3. Pathogenetic mechanisms that may be involved in the etiology of essential hypertension (arrow signifies "increase" or "elevation" in). (Adapted from Kaplan.[24] Reprinted from *Modern Medicine*© The New York Times Company, Inc.)

That genetic mechanisms may indirectly control blood pressure is strongly suggested by animal studies which demonstrate a high heritability for blood pressure. Selection studies have shown that "spontaneous" differences in blood pressure may readily be selected for[25] and that more than one gene is involved.[26] The evidence for a genetic basis for hypertension in man is both direct and indirect: a single pleiotropic gene or closely linked autosomal dominants have been convincingly shown to be responsible for both hypertension and brachydactyly.[27] While single-gene hypotheses have appeared in the past,[28] the modern consensus is that hypertension has a polygenic basis.[29,30] Figure 4 summarizes data which compare the frequency of elevated blood pressure among relatives of those with hypertension.[31]

In general, the systolic and diastolic indices used to measure hypertension rise with age and body weight in populations at risk for hypertension.[32] Strong exogenous factors associated with high blood pressure in these populations include sodium intake, dietary fat and animal protein. These factors combine to make any estimation of "hypertension" based on blood pressure alone an exceedingly difficult undertaking. Note that the abscissal scales of Figure 4 are different for diastolic and systolic blood pressures (parts A and B), and that the diastolic scale terminates at 140 mg of mercury while the systolic one reaches 210 mg. Figure 4C reflects the lack of distinctness between the three curves and their

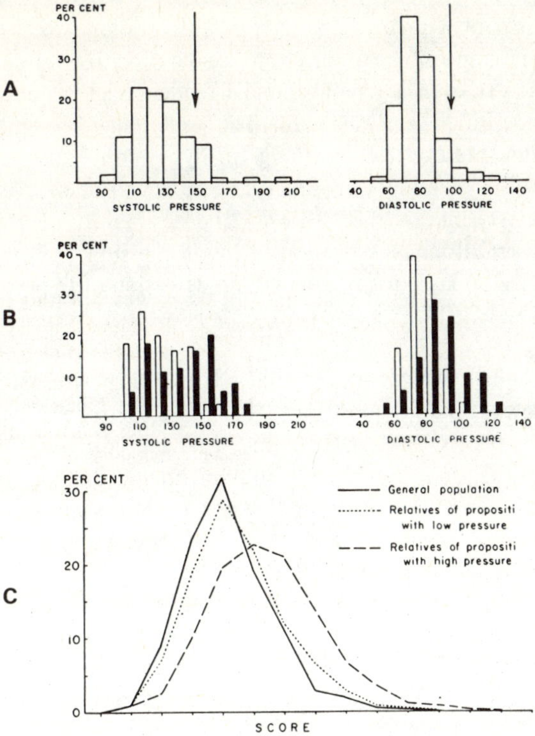

Fig. 4. Arterial blood pressures. (A) Sample of 277 women, 30-39 years old. *The arrows point to the pressures often used to separate groups with normal and high blood pressure.* (B) Forty-six female relatives of propositi with low pressures (controls, *light columns*) as compared with 41 female relatives of propositi with high pressures (hypertensives, *dark columns*), ages 30-39 years. (C) Frequency distributions of diastolic pressures for 867 persons from the general population, 371 relatives of controls and 1,062 relatives of hypertensives; males and females, 10-79 years old. Since different age groups as well as both sexes have different mean pressures, the curves are adjusted for age and sex. (From Hamilton et al.[31])

considerable overlap. The most distinct, however, is that drawn for the relatives of patients with high blood pressure. In the case of continuous variables correlated with multifactorial inheritance such as these, how do we define the diseased state? When does high blood pressure become hypertension? At [150 systolic/100 diastolic]? At what age or in which race? And what is mild or borderline hypertension? Even if we do define it, we still cannot predict with any reliable degree of accuracy those individuals who will develop hypertension within a given family.

The absence of a precisely known genetic etiology for hypertension thus makes it impossible to give precise empiric risks to relatives of hypertensives; yet even a general familial tendency allows at-risk individuals to be identified early in life. The real issues in embarking on population-wide prescriptive screening for hypertensive disease, however, have to do with detecting individuals *not* known to be at higher risk for hypertension. At stake is the "efficacy and desirability of detecting and treating mild symptomless elevation of blood pressure."[32] Just what are the mechanisms available for treatment and detection of hypertension?

Therapy

A large number of agents of several pharmacologic classes exist which effectively lower blood pressure. There are peripheral vasodilators, beta-blocking agents and potassium-conserving drugs.[32,33] General hygienic measures such as reducing sodium intake, dieting, etc. are too well known to review here. As with diabetes it is important to identify the principal pathologic sequelae and to ask if therapeutic intervention in hypertension has a demonstrable effect.

The specific pathologies associated with hypertension are in order of causal association: (1) arterial disease, especially atheroma or nodular arteriosclerosis, (2) Charcot-Bouchard aneurysms (rupture of the minute cerebral arteries), (3) fibrinoid necrosis of small arteries and arterioles (caused by malignant hypertension).[34] Arterial disease, as manifested by ischemic heart disease, has been shown by the Framingham study to be approximately twice the expected incidence in persons with definite hypertension (159/95).[35]

While there is some evidence that reducing blood pressure in hypertensives reduces the incidence of strokes or other Charcot-Bouchard phenomena,[32] according to some researchers there is little evidence that it reduces the frequency or severity of heart attacks.[32,36] Others contest that treatment is in fact "ineffective" in preventing cardiovascular complications,[37] or in reducing "general complications"[38]; but there is universal agreement that early institution of treatment would be necessary to ameliorate the major consequences. Indeed, since it is easier to restore "normal" blood pressure in young adults (<20 years) than in older ones (>35 years), and since childhood elevated blood pressure is statistically associated with later values, it has been suggested that screening and treatment be started in mildly hypertensive young adults and children.[38]

Assuming that sufficient means exist to detect the prehypertensive adult and incipient hypertensive child (see below under "Detection"), the question still remains whether such screening has a therapeutic rationale. As a working principle, we agree with the anonymous editorial which recently advocated: "The earlier the physician starts to treat hypertension, and the milder [its] degree, the greater is his responsibility to ensure that treatment is justifiable."[38]

The authors of the most recent study of the effects of lowering blood pressure in moderately hypertensive individuals (100 to 120 mm Hg) reported entirely inconclusive results.[39] Similarly, the author of a review of systemic hypertension in children concluded that "there is little information about the efficacy, side effects, or metabolism of the antihypertensive drugs in children of various ages."[40] A fair evaluation of the actions predicated on this type of information appears to us to be that it would be "unwise . . . to embark on clinical trials of the treatment of marginal hypertension in childhood with drugs."[38] We are less sure of the contraindications for instituting therapy in the moderately hypertensive adult, but we must reject the rationale for the notion of mass screening – in the face of present ignorance – expressed by the former Secretary of Health, Education and Welfare, Elliot Richardson:

> We have no dramatic breakthrough in hypertension, yet . . . I am convinced that we have enough knowledge to make a resolution to put [screening] into practice throughout our country. During the decade of the 1970's, physicians *are going to become* more proficient than before in knowing when and how to treat and detect hypertension.[36] (italics ours)

In our view, mass hypertension screening should be conducted on a provisional basis, while screening of high-risk groups, especially young adult blacks, should be encouraged.

Detection

In spite of the statement that no large series has yet demonstrated the utility of various diagnostic tests for revealing the etiology of persistent hypertension,[40] the myth persists that a single sitting or supine blood pressure measurement taken independent of follow-up is all that is needed for a definitive diagnosis. Among the most pressing diagnostic needs is some means of distinguishing labile from essential hypertension. A new means of distinguishing between these two disorders has been proposed, using the presence of increased levels of dopamine-beta-hydroxylase as an indicator.[41] Although such a marker would undoubtedly lead to a more efficient method for diagnosing persons at risk for developing hypertension, the developer of the test cautions that we will "need a 20 year study to see if all labiles, or only certain ones, will convert to essential hypertension."[41]

With regard to a specific carrier detection test for hypertension, one may consider the use of a pressor, ie a stimulus used to increase the activity of some physiologic function, here vasomotor activity. It has been suggested that reactions to a cold pressor may be employed to detect potential essential hypertensives. One arm is submerged in cold water while the resulting degree and rate of elevation in blood pressure are measured in the other arm. The reliability of this test, however, is doubtful.[42]

In sum, there is as yet no reliable test for identifying the prehypertensive; and according to two researchers, there is a pressing need to find the antecedents to hypertension early in life.[29] This situation leaves us with the vexing question raised elsewhere in this volume (see papers by Lappé and Roblin; Powledge; and Murray), as to whether or not large-scale *research* screens are justifiable, especially in children. The rationale of such screening, as well as that to detect the presymptomatic adult, rests in the main on our future conclusions regarding the efficacy of treatments for moderate hypertension, and the ultimate impact on reducing the estimated 60,000 deaths from hypertension-associated disease yearly.[34] We also note that while mass screening seems indicated in view of the large (approximately 40%) proportion of undetected cases,[37,43] in practice as few as 8% of the newly detected cases return for follow-up.[44] This points to the need for adequate education programs, as well as community involvement. While mass screening has been done recently (Baldwin City, Ga. National Health Survey; Alameda City Blood Pressure Survey; Peoples Gas Co. [Chicago] ; Family Planning Clinics [Washington, D. C.] ; Health Department [New Orleans] ; and Maryland),[44] there are no data on the long-term benefits *on a population-wide scale* as weighed against possible medical or psychosocial risks or hazards of early intervention. There are reports of "unnecessary referrals" and "worry" following hypertension screening[44]; and in the absence of reliable evidence that the clinical expression of prehypertension can be delayed or prevented,[39] we believe it would be premature to institute such programs on a mass scale. The need to improve the efficacy of hypertension screening programs has been recognized by at least one state subcommittee.[45] [Guidelines are available from Dr. S. B. Garbus; Louisiana State University Medical Center, 1542 Tulane Avenue, New Orleans, La. 70112.]

Neural Tube Defects

The two principal neural tube defects are anencephaly and spina bifida. Anencephaly is characterized by the absence of the bones of the cranial vault and defective development of the cerebellar and cerebral hemispheres. A reasonable hypothesis for its origin is that embryologically, the medullary plate associated with the neural tube and, later, the spinal cord does not rise and close over anteriorly, so that what should be a canal becomes a groove. Approximately 1-3 per 1,000 births are currently anencephalic in the U.S. Caucasian population. This incidence may increase with maternal age, and it occurs more often among female neonates than males.[46-48] Spina bifida, on the other hand, most probably results from nonclosure of a posterior portion of the neural plate. This produces an open neural tube in more or less extensive regions of the spinal column and, later, an open vertebral canal.

While anencephaly is always lethal, treated spina bifida usually is not, depending upon the extent and site of the defect. Spina bifida is a phenotypically variable condition, and is the most common malformation of the spinal cord and vertebral column. Of all such defects, 0.5% occur in the lumbar region of the spine, 12% are lumbrosacral and 27% sacral. In spina bifida occulta, no neurologic symptoms may occur, but children who have difficulty learning to walk or a clumsy gait and enuresis or sphincter trouble may harbor the defect. Often a fistula on the back discharges cerebrospinal fluid, or there is only a dimple in overlying skin denoting the spot where a fistula has closed. Anencephaly and spina bifida may occur together, and there are kinships with both conditions represented in varying degrees of severity. Relatives of defective children may have subtle spinal defects,[49] brought to light only by x rays of the lower spine in individuals with no clinical manifestations.

Is it possible that anencephaly and spina bifida are parts of a continuum such that they share a single hereditary base? Both represent the absence or incompleteness of embryonic ectodermal neural tubular movements, and both can in no way be assigned to simple "mendelizing" genetic factors, as we will discuss below. While it has been argued that there may be no genetic basis for anencephaly and spina bifida,[48] we wish to review the evidence.

Evidence for a Polygenic Etiology

The evidence that there is a genetic basis underlying the expression of neural tube defects has accrued over the last ten years. In 1960, almost 1,100 cases were reviewed with an overall recurrence rate in sibs born after the first index case of 4.6%. However, the authors of this study concluded that "the recurrence of these anomalies in sibships is as likely to be due to persistence or recurrence of environmental factors as to a common genetic inheritance."[49] It is difficult to deduce genetic mechanisms from the range of estimates for sib recurrence rates which vary from 2.7% to 6.1%; however, a calculation of the incidence of offspring of adults affected with spina bifida has recently become possible. In a sample of 215 survivors Carter and Evans found that the risk to offspring of neural tube defect is 3% (or about 30 times the expected incidence).[50] This proportion is comparable to sib recurrence rates,[cf 51] and is independent of sex of parent, reducing the likelihood that maternal factors play a determining role in neural tube defects.[52] These authors were also forced to conclude, however, that in the aggregate, data on recurrence rates do *not* help distinguish between polygenic or other modes of inheritance (eg modified monogenic).

We may conclude that while a polygenic mode of inheritance cannot be excluded from these studies, there is as yet no overwhelmingly convincing data for its acceptance. The relevance of this conclusion is heightened by the observation that while variable genetic susceptibility to environmental components is a possible explanation, the most hopeful hypothesis (with regard to interventions) is that of environmental variables.[51] (For example, see a recent symposium held in St. Jovite, Quebec on June 14, 1973 which reviewed the evidence for a causal relationship between belighted potatoes and spinal cord defects [*Teratology, 8*:317-361, 1973].) Discordant anencephaly in monozygotic twins further undermines the genetic hypothesis.

Potential Therapies

At this stage of our ignorance about the possible teratologic mechanisms leading to neural tube defects, "therapies" must be instituted after the fact, in contrast to the general philosophy of prescriptive screening for preemptive intervention. Dietary restriction of potatoes, for example, has been disputed as an effective means of reducing the incidence of anencephaly. Prognosis is so uniformly negative and conclusive in anencephaly as to lead us to conclude that "early intervention" in the form of abortion is now the only real "therapeutic" option. The "therapeutic" problem of anencephaly is thus largely one of identifying at-risk kindreds and effecting an early detection of affected fetuses. This will be considered below. The question of treatment for spina bifida, especially where it is complicated by myelomeningocele, is a knotty one. Lorber has reviewed the question of universal treatment for spina bifida cystica in light of the often predictably poor quality of life which current surgical corrective procedures offer.[53] As a result of treating 524 unselected cases, he concluded that it is possible to forecast the minimum degree of future handicap if surgery is performed, and that selection of cases for surgery should be based on some set of agreed-upon criteria. Complete exploration of this complex topic is beyond the scope of the present manuscript.

For the purposes of a discussion of screening, the relevant question is whether or not any indices of either spina bifida cystica or anencephaly can be used to meaningfully anticipate the birth of affected children. For example, if it were possible to make a diagnosis in utero of spina bifida *and* if some variant of Lorber's criteria could be applied to the fetus, an early decision to terminate pregnancy might be facilitated in some cases.[53] At some later time, the question of fetal surgery might be entertained. Now, it is likely that the entire question of screening for neural tube defects rests on their detection in utero, since abortion is now and is likely to continue to be the only option for parents facing the prospect of a severely affected offspring.

Detection

Four recent developments have afforded opportunities for early detection of affected fetuses, especially in high-risk sibships. The first is applicable to either condition, but will have greatest value for estimating the degree of severity of spina bifida. It entails visual observation of the fetus in situ through a fiber optic device. A surgical endoamnioscope makes this possible since it provides an $80^\circ \pm 5^\circ$ field of view. This new endoamnioscope permits the visualization of fetal tissue with direct vision under general or local anesthesia through a small 2-inch-long laparotomy. Sonar placentography is first employed to localize the placenta, in preparation for the subsequent insertion of the endoamnioscope. Apparently minimal complications accompany use of this instrument (Fig. 5) when it is employed as directed by its developers, Valenti and Quint.[54,55]

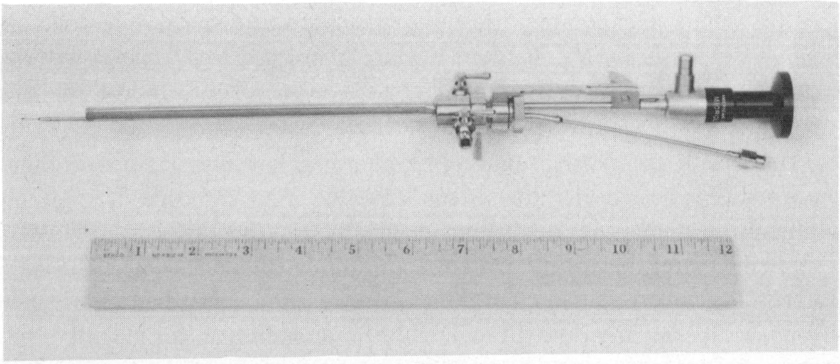

Fig. 5. The endoamnioscope of Valenti and Quint[54,55]; its total cost approximates $1,000 and it allows the viewing and biopsy of fetal tissue.

However, it has been shown that some amniotic membrane may be trapped in the incision when the amnioscope is withdrawn (Valenti, personal communication).

A second development permits antenatal detection of one class of defect, anencephaly. In using ultrasound to localize the placenta, it has been recognized that the fetal head gives a distinct echo. Four British investigators first utilized this fact in 1972 in diagnosing an anencephalic fetus at 17 weeks in a woman who had taken clomiphene (examination was done to exclude multiple pregnancy).[56] Midtrimester abortion was successfully performed after confirmation of the ultrasound readings at weekly intervals for two weeks. The authors recommend this screening procedure for all women who have previously had a baby with spina bifida or an anencephalic fetus.[56]

The third opportunity for detection of either anencephaly or spina bifida has been enhanced by the development of technical and biochemical procedures for sampling and assaying the amniotic fluid. Several developments have been made in the early 1970s which greatly increase the possibilities of success. Of the three diagnostic possibilities visualized in early 1972 – (1) a fortuitous biochemical abnormality, (2) a changed concentration of neural tissue metabolites, or (3) a changed concentration of other metabolites – essentially all have come to fruition. As an example of the second, 5-hydroxyindole (5-HIAA) is present in decreased amounts in the amniotic fluids of pregnancies where the fetus has a malformation of the central nervous system.[57] This metabolite appears to offer the possibility of distinguishing between severely and mildly affected spina bifida fetuses, since a decrease in 5-HIAA is thought to occur only where there is a defect severe enough to involve kidney function. As an example of the third, Emery and Burt reported increased amounts of specific amino acids in amniotic fluid taps that fortuitously were done on pregnancies with central nervous system abnormalities.[58] The question remains, however, whether such increases were specific indices of the abnormality in question or reflections of fetal distress.

The fourth and most promising development in detecting neural tube abnormalities has been the recent (1973) discovery that a protein (alpha-fetoprotein), presumably produced by the fetal liver, is markedly increased in pregnancies at risk for spina bifida or anencephaly.[59] Since the first discovery, others have shown that an increased level of this substance in the amniotic fluid is a specific indicator for neural tube defects. Detection may be done as early as 13 weeks' gestation, allowing uneventful termination of pregnancy.[60]

Interestingly, in this last study alpha-fetoprotein *alone* was used in one case as the determinant, since neither ultrasound nor x ray gave confirmatory readings. The obvious moral question posed by the chance of aborting false-positives on this basis alone must be confronted. Perhaps amnioscopy can be used in the future as a means of anatomically corroborating such ambiguous findings and for determining the degree of prospective neural tube defect.* In the authors' view, the principal value of these technics is to allow women who might not have considered a second pregnancy at 5%-10% risk for neural tube defect, to attempt another child.[60]

Were this all that could be said about prenatal diagnosis for these often assuredly severe defects, we would be unjustified in including this discussion in our paper. However, the recent finding of Brock et al[61] that *maternal* serum contains raised levels of alpha-fetoprotein in the presence of anterior neural tube defective fetuses, affords a prospective test for anencephaly. They do strongly urge though that maternal serum not be used alone in diagnosing the condition, since other conditions generate raised alpha-fetoprotein levels. (We are aware of at least five physiologic states in which this is the case, eg uremia, leukemia, Hodgkin disease, x irradiation and, in particular, the hepatocellular carcinomas cited by Brock.)

The significance of this study in Brock's words is "that it raises the possibility of screening pregnancies through a determination made on a small amount of blood."[61] By inference this could be considered an open invitation to mass screening for neural tube defects. We believe that, although the current state of the art militates against widespread application, at-risk families should be afforded this option, and reevaluation should be periodically done to assess further the test's applicability and accuracy.

Conclusions and Summary

In concluding it would be well to review the criteria that are generally recognized as prerequisites for screening and to determine how well each of the three types of conditions we have studied meet them. Paraphrasing Wilson and Jungner,[5] we can identify these general principles in screening:

1. The disorder to be screened must be an important health problem.
2. Its etiology must be reasonably well known.

---

*Adequate consideration of the latitude of subjective interpretation of the "burden" imposed by neural tube defects should be used in applying these technics to ensure that parents are under no psychologic pressure to abort.

3. It must have a recognizable presymptomatic phase and an understandable natural history.
4. It must be treatable, preferably in its early stages.
5. Sensitive tests must exist for distinguishing the condition from "normal" or from subclinical states of the disorder.
6. There must be a cut-off point between those found to need or not to need treatment.
7. It must be cost-effective to screen at the time and in the population identified as suitable.

(We note parenthetically that there are other dimensions to validating screening programs: these have been presented by members of the Genetics Group of the Institute of Society, Ethics and Life Sciences.[62])

Each of the conditions chosen for discussion can be said to represent a significant health problem or pose substantial psychologic and social burdens on individuals and families (eg spina bifida and anencephaly). In each of the conditions discussed, however, the etiology is only sketchily known and a polygenic basis for its inheritance is only broadly inferred. However, we do not believe that such an omission in our understanding disqualifies these disorders from consideration. *In our view the principal value of discerning a polygenic basis for the inheritance of a disorder or disease is to enable more accurate identification of persons at increased risk, and to infer important conclusions regarding its pathogenesis and likely susceptibility to treatment.* With the exception of the neural tube defects, the disorders we have considered have a theoretic presymptomatic stage, but precise means of delimiting this period are not yet available. Nevertheless, both diabetes and hypertension are presaged by *some* identifying physiologic aberration, eg a decreased tolerance to glucose following cortisone sensitization or an alteration in the level of dopamine-beta-hydroxylase. More precise and universally applicable means of detection seem likely in the future; however, the very polygenic nature of the etiology of these conditions makes fulfillment of precise discrimination of incipient disease from normal variability exceedingly difficult.

While a modicum of therapeutic benefit is consistently reported for virtually any method which restores normal clinical readings in diabetes (urinary blood sugar "O") or hypertension ("normal" blood pressure, eg less than 100 mm Hg), the absence of a consensus concerning the basic defect in each disorder renders development of other than symptom-dependent therapeutic modalities highly uncertain. This impasse makes the distinction of treatment needs of the normal but presymptomatic person from those of the symptomatic but preclinical person ambiguous. A foreseeable consequence is that substantial numbers of "normal" individuals will have to be treated to assure that presymptomatic individuals receive optimal preemptive care. As others have emphasized, this situation poses major eithical and social questions not commonly encountered in other forms of genetic screening where "presumptive" diagnoses can usually be made with near certainty, thereby minimizing the problem of treating the false-positive.

Mass screening for neural tube defects on the basis of maternal serum (rather than intraamniotic) determinations of the presence of alpha-fetoprotein must, of course, be followed by conclusive corroborations of the status of the fetus, since many conditions may produce false-positive signs. Ultrasound, x ray and, in the future, amnioscopy promise to make this diagnosis fail-safe, but until then each pregnancy will have to be handled individually with considerable technical back-up. Consequently, mass screening for this condition is in the not-too-distant future, but not currently a reasonable prospect until the commitment of follow-up materials and personnel are made. We believe that the incidence and severity of both classes of neural tube defects warrant a major commitment to considering their screening; but some criteria must be set up to ensure that appropriate guidelines exist (eg the appropriate identification of gradations of severity for spina bifida cystica) so that only marginally impaired, or near normal individuals will not be automatically discarded with those whose prospective quality of life is assessed to be severely compromised.[63] We note that almost 50% of apparently *normal* children have minor spinal cord abnormalities which sophisticated technics might well detect in utero.

In sum, the major categories of human disability subsumed under "diabetes mellitus" and "hypertension" point up the urgent need to mobilize resources to anticipate their development in individuals. The likely polygenic basis for their expression, however, confounds simple analysis of the desirability of instituting mass screening for presymptomatic individuals. Until more precise information about the specific causes of these disabilities is available, coupled with good data on the prognosis of those treated early, the presymptomatic screening for these conditions will remain at an experimental stage, and should be presented as such.

Acknowledgment

The authors gratefully acknowledge the assistance of Robert Murray, Jr., M.D. in preparing sections of this manuscript.

References

1. Murphy, E. A.: Some difficulties in the investigation of genetic factors in coronary artery disease. *Canad. Med. J., 7*:1181, 1967.
2. Murphy, E. A.: Genetic and hematologic factors in venous thrombosis. *Milbank Med. Fund Quart.*, suppl. 2:71, 1972.
3. Carter, C. O.: Multifactorial genetic disease. *Hosp. Pract.*, May, 1970, p. 45.
4. Herskowitz, I.: *Principles of Genetics.* New York:Macmillan Publishing Co., 1973.
5. Wilson, M. C. and Jungner, G.: *Principles and Practice of Screening for Disease.* Geneva:World Health Organization, 1968.
6. Neel, J., Fajans, S., Conn, J. and Davidson, R.: Diabetes mellitus. In *Genetics and Epidemiology of Chronic Diseases,* publ. 1163, Department of Health, Education and Welfare, Public Health Service, 1965, p. 105.
7. Darlow, J. M., Smith, C. and Duncan, L. J. P.: A statistical and genetical study of diabetes. *Ann. Hum. Genet., 37*:157, 1973.
8. Rimoin, D. L.: Inheritance in diabetes mellitus. *Med. Clin. N. Amer., 55*:807-819, 1971.
9. Pincus, G. and White, P.: On the inheritance of diabetes mellitus, I. An analysis of 675 family histories. *Amer. J. Med. Sci., 186*:1, 1933.
10. Steinberg, A.: Genetics of diabetes mellitus: A review. *Ann. N. Y. Acad. Sci., 82*:197, 1959.
11. Steinberg, A.: Genetics and diabetes. In *On the Nature and Treatment of Diabetes.* Excerpta Medica International Congress Series 83, 1965.
12. Mimura, G. and Miyao, S.: Heredity and constitutions of diabetes mellitus. *Bull. Res. Inst. Diathetic Med. Kumamoto Univ., 12*:1, 1962.
13. Pavel, I. and Pieptea, R.: Etude sur la diabete hereditaire au cours de 3 et 4 generations successives. *Diabetologia, 2*:281, 1966.
14. Simpson, N.: Multifactorial inheritance: A possible hypothesis for diabetes. *Diabetes, 13*:462, 1964.
15. Penrose, L. and Watson, E.: A sex-linked tendency in familial diabetics. *Proc. Amer. Diabetes Assoc., 5*:165, 1945.
16. Aronberg, A., Larsson, T. and Jung, J.: Diabetes in Sweden: A clinicostatistical, epidemiological and genetic study of hospital patients and death certificates. *Acta Med. Scand., 477*:126, 1967.
17. Rimoin, D.: Genetics of diabetes mellitus. *Diabetes, 16*:346, 1967.
18. Simpson, N.: Multifactorial inheritance: A possible hypothesis for diabetes. *Diabetes, 13*:462, 1964.
19. Weil, W.: Juvenile diabetes mellitus. In Bergsma, D. (ed.): *Birth Defects: Atlas and Compendium.* Baltimore:Williams and Wilkins, (for The National Foundation – March of Dimes), 1973.
20. Butterfield, W. J. H.: Diabetes mellitus. In *Screening in Medical Care.* New York:Oxford Univeristy Press, 1968, pp. 65-80.
21. Whichelow, M. J., Wigglesworth, A., Cox, B. D. et al: Critical analysis of blood sugar measurements in diabetes detection and diagnosis. *Diabetes, 16*:4, 1967.
22. Walsh, G. H., O'Regan, J. and O'Sullivan, D. J.: Effect of different periods of fasting on oral glucose tolerance. *Brit. Med. J., 2*:691-693, 1973.
23. Robinson, S. K.: The campaign to combat essential hypertension. *JAMA, 233*:1286, 1973.

24. Kaplan, N. M.: The puzzle of essential hypertension. *Mod. Med.*, April 2, 1973, pp. 26-30.
25. Dupont, J., Dupont, J. C., Froment, A. et al: Selection of three strains of rats with spontaneously different levels of blood pressure. *Biomedicine, 19*:36-41, 1973.
26. Hansen, C. T.: The genetic regulation of blood pressure in the rat. In *Genetics 74* (suppl. 2, part 2), Proceedings XIII International Congress of Genetics, Berkeley, Calif. June, 1973, p. 106.
27. Bilginturan, N., Zilelli, S., Karacadag, S. and Pirnar, T.: Hereditary brachydactyly associated with hypertension. *J. Med. Gen., 10*:253-259, 1973.
28. Platt, R.: Essential hypertension: Incidence, course, and heredity. *Ann. Intern. Med., 55*:1-11, 1961.
29. Miall, W. E. and Oldham, P. D.: The hereditary factor in arterial blood pressure. *Brit. Med. J., 1*:75-79, 1963.
30. Page, L. B. and Sidd, J. J.: Medical management of primary hypertension. *N. Eng. J. Med., 287*:960-967; 1018-1023, 1972.
31. Hamilton, M., Pickering, G., Roberts, J. and Sowry, G.: Aetiology of essential hypertension 4. Role of inheritance. *Clin. Sci., 13*:273, 1954.
32. Anonymous: Hypertension up-to-date. *Lancet, 2*:951-952, 1973.
33. Aagard, G. N.: The management of hypertension. *JAMA, 224*:329-332, 1973.
34. Pickering, G.: Hypertension: Definitions, natural histories and consequences. *Amer. J. Med., 52*:570-583, 1972.
35. Kannel, W. and Gordon, T. (eds.): *Framingham Study*. Section 27. Washington: U.S., Superintend. of Documents No. HE 20,3002; F84/Sec. 27, Govt. Prtg. Off. 1740-0320, 1971.
36. Cooper, T.: The national hypertension program. *J. Amer. Pharm. Assoc., NS-13*:135-138, 1973.
37. Freis, E. D.: Hypertension: A challenge in preventive cardiology. *Circulation, 47*:1-2, 1973.
38. Anonymous: Detection of hypertension in childhood. *Brit. Med. J., 2*:365-366, 1973.
39. Anonymous: Control of moderately raised blood pressure. *Brit. Med. J., 2*:434-436, 1973.
40. Loggie, J. M. H.: Systemic hypertension in children, *Pediat. Clin. N. Amer., 18*:1273-1309, 1971.
41. Anonymous: Enzyme tag for the pressure-prone? *Medical World News,* Sept. 14, 1973, pp. 71-72.
42. *Hypertension Bulletins,* Ciba Pharmaceuticals. Summit, N. J.:International Medical Press, 1973.
43. Wilber, J. A.: The problem of undetected and untreated hypertension in the community. *Bull. N. Y. Acad. Med., 49*:510-520, 1973.
44. Kilcoyne, M. M.: Hypertension and heart disease in the urban community. *Bull. N. Y. Acad. Med., 49*:501-509, 1973.
45. Saunders, E.: Screening for hypertension. *Maryland Med. J., 22*:32-34, 1973.
46. Woolf, C.: Stillbirth and parental age. *Obstet. Gynec., 26*:1, 1965.
47. Penrose, L.: Maternal age, order of birth and developmental abnormalities. *J. Ment. Sci., 85*:1141, 1939 (Table).
48. Janerich, D. T.: Anencephaly and maternal age. *Amer. J. Epidemiol., 95*:319-326, 1972.

49. Yen, S. and MacMahon, B.: Genetics of anencephaly and spina bifida? *Lancet, 2*:623-626, 1968.
50. Carter, C. O. and Evans, K.: Children of adult survivors with spina bifida cystica. *Lancet, 2*:924-926, 1973.
51. Anonymous: Epidemics of anencephaly and spina bifida. *Lancet, 1*:689-900, 1971.
52. Janerich, D. T.: Maternal age and spina bifida: Longitudinal versus cross-sectional analysis. *Amer. J. Epidemiol., 96*:389-395, 1973.
53. Lorber, J.: Results of treatment of myelomeningocele. *Dev. Med. Child. Neurol., 13*:279-303, 1971.
54. Valenti, C.: Endoamnioscopy and fetal biopsy: A new technique. *Amer. J. Obstet. Gynec., 114*:561, 1972.
55. Valenti, C.: Antenatal detection of hemoglobinopathies. *Amer. J. Obstet. Gynec., 115*:851, 1973.
56. Campbell, S., Holt, E. M., Johnstone, F. D. and May, P.: Anencephaly: Early ultrasonic diagnosis and active management. *Lancet, 2*:1226-1227, 1972.
57. Emery, A. E. H., Eccleston, D., Scrimgeour, J. B. and Johnstone, M.: Amniotic fluid composition in malformations of the central nervous system. *J. Obstet. Gynaec. Brit. Comm., 79*:154-158, 1972.
58. Emery, A. E. H. and Burt, D.: Aminoacid composition of amniotic fluid in central nervous system malformations. *Lancet, 1*:970-971, 1973.
59. Brock, D. J. H. and Sutcliffe, R. G.: Alpha-fetoprotein in the antenatal diagnosis of anencephaly and spina bifida. *Lancet, 2*:197-199, 1972.
60. Allan, L. D., Donald, I., Ferguson-Smith, M. A. et al: Amniotic-fluid alpha-fetoprotein in the antenatal diagnosis of spina bifida. *Lancet, 2*:522-525, 1973.
61. Brock, D. J. H., Bolton, A. E. and Monaghan, J. M.: Prenatal diagnosis of anencephaly through maternal serum-alphafetoprotein measurement. *Lancet, 2*:923-924, 1973.
62. Genetics Group of the Institute of Society, Ethics and Life Sciences: Ethical and social issues in screening for human genetic disease. *N. Eng. J. Med., 286*:1129-1132, 1972.
63. Anonymous: The spinal cord in spina bifida. *Lancet, 2*:830-831, 1973.

Chromosomal Screening of Human Populations

A Bioethical Prospectus

William J. Mellman, M.D.

A remarkable series of observations has been made in the past 15 years about chromosome variation in human populations. In the first years of this period of discovery, most human biologists certainly did not expect the degree of variation that was revealed. Despite the large amount of scientific interest generated by these discoveries, inadequate attention may have been paid to the potential social implications of results of human population cytogenetic studies. Just as with screening programs for biochemical genetic diseases, chromosomal screening is in the "gray zone" between health care and genetic research. For this reason, both the experimental goals and the ethical, psychologic and sociomedical problems faced need to be carefully scrutinized by both human geneticists and the public who participate in population surveys for chromosome disorders.

This paper surveys the spectrum of information already available about human cytogenetics and concludes that, on the basis of what we have already discovered, those who propose future population studies to learn more about human chromosome variation must start asking different questions about different types of chromosome deviations. The information to be sought will have differing social impacts, and consequently individualized strategies will need to be employed in acquiring the various data. Chromosome studies will increasingly require extensive forays into human populations; as with mass genetic screening, this will consequently focus attention on the need for greater social responsibility among those who operate such programs.

William J. Mellman, M.D., *Professor and Chairman, Department of Human Genetics, University of Pennsylvania School of Medicine, Philadelphia.*

What do we know about the cytogenetics of human populations?

In the late 1950s, technics were developed that permitted chromosomal analysis of the peripheral blood leukocytes of relatively large numbers of individuals in selected populations. Because this has been and still is a manual procedure, the total number of individuals studied by a single laboratory has been limited. Promises of automated methods are yet unfulfilled despite the serious efforts of a highly talented group of laboratories.[1-3] Because the initial discoveries of gross human chromosomal deviations were in persons who were either mentally retarded or physically malformed, or persons who evidenced disorders of sexual differentiation or development, or who suffered from malignancy (leukemia specifically)[4] these have been the special groups most extensively surveyed. The individuals studied were participants exclusively because of their clinical problems, and hence were studied as part of the established health evaluation process.

In the early 1960s a group in Edinburgh established the value of moving beyond the boundaries of traditional medical evaluation. Their classic work on the long-term effects in lymphocyte chromosomes of x-irradiation used in the treatment of ankylosing spondylitis[5] was followed by surveys of workers with industrial exposure to irradiation and toxic substances such as benzene and mercurials.[6] The need for comparison with "control" adult populations was recognized by this group and relatively limited numbers of healthy subjects chosen at random from the rolls of family practitioners were examined.

The study of 207 males and 231 females reported in 1966[7] stands as one of the largest recorded "normal" adult studies. This survey and supplemental data from less "normal" groups of subjects have revealed that structural abnormalities of chromosomes occur in about 3 per 1,000 individuals of the population.[6] The limited size of surveyed adult populations does not allow for any precision of this estimate. Nonetheless, these adult data have been extremely useful to investigators who have examined random newborn populations.

Most of the attention paid to adult populations, in addition to those special groups already cited, has been to the socially deviant. Jacobs et al[8,9] as well as Casey et al[10] reported an unusually high incidence of XYY individuals among males in British maximum-security hospitals. Court-Brown concluded from his analysis of the information on XYY available in 1968 that the problem of interpreting the existing data could be solved by identification of XYY males at birth and surveillance from birth onward.[11]

What have we learned from studies of newborn populations?

The overwhelming bulk of data acquired from unselected human populations has come from chromosomal surveys of liveborn hospital births. In 1970 an accounting was made of the five largest surveys in progress. Although a total of 16,647 infants had been analyzed at that time, it was pointed out then that three surveys were still in progress and estimated that information on 14,000 additional infants per year would be obtained.

Table 1 summarizes the frequency of chromosomal abnormalities detected in these pooled data.

The chromosomes of approximately 1 in 200 newborns display a major chromosomal variation, either a structural rearrangement or a deviation in the number of autosomes or sex chromosomes (ie chromosome aneuploidy).

If currently available technics for staining chromosomes had been employed in these surveys, a remarkable number of other, more subtle variations would have been detected. How these variants affect the individuals in whom they are found is uncertain at the present time.[12,13] The same must be said for the majority of the structural rearrangements revealed in these populations by conventional staining methods, especially in view of the likelihood that the frequency of structural rearrangements in healthy adult populations may be similar to that of newborns.

Autosomal aneuploidy in newborn infants has been observed almost exclusively in those with recognizable clinical syndromes (eg mongolism or trisomy 18 syndrome).

The sex chromosome aneuploidies command our special attention since they comprise nearly one-half of the total deviations detected in newborn chromosomal surveys, specifically, 2.81/1000 male births and 1.25/1000 female births. As seen in Table 2 there are five types of sex chromosome aneuploidy which predominate in newborn populations.

Table 1. Summary of Neonatal Chromosome Surveys

Total Newborn Infants	16,647
Male	11,039
Female	5,608
Structural rearrangements/1,000 live births	1.80
Autosomal aneuploidy/1,000 live births	1.08
Sex chromosome aneuploidy/1,000 male live births	2.81
Sex chromosome aneuploidy/1,000 female live births	1.25
Total abnormalities/1,000 live births	**4.91**

Table 2. Frequency of Specific Sex Chromosome Aneuploidies in Newborn Surveys

XYY	1.5/1,000 males
XXY	1.2/1,000 males
XXX	1.1/1,000 females
XO	0.2/1,000 females
XX	0.1/1,000 males

The XO female has a clinically recognizable phenotype,[14] and the XX male, despite his often profound difficulties,[15] occurs at such a low frequency that we can ignore these two conditions for purposes of this discussion.

There would appear to be no currently defined medical indication for screening populations to detect either autosomal aneuploidy or structural rearrangements. As already stated, individuals with autosomal aneuploidy are clinically identifiable in the absence of prior chromosomal detection, and the structural rearrangements, at least at a societal level, cannot be categorized as a health concern. The sex chromosome aneuploidies may be a different situation. Should we be screening populations more actively to detect XYY, XXY and XXX individuals, and if so, what social issues are generated by such proposed programs?

How valid are newborn frequencies as estimates of population incidences?

The validity of newborn frequencies is a critical question since our knowledge of the chromosomal constitution of the general population is almost exclusively limited to this age group.

The goals of newborn chromosomal screening up to now have been clearly of a research nature – to establish the frequency of specific chromosomal abnormalities and to determine their phenotypic manifestations. However, these newborn frequencies can only be used as first approximations when compared with special groups, such as socially deviant adult populations. Although Court-Brown urged the study of newborn populations to detect XYY babies, who would then be observed during development for evidence of deviant behavior, he and other epidemiologists have emphasized the fallacy of using newborns as references for populations of other ages.[16,17] The distinction has been made between *incidence,* defined as rate of occurrence at birth, and *prevalence,* defined as the number of cases in various age groups in a population at a given point in time.[18] A comparison of the frequencies of chromosomal abnormalities in newborn populations with those in deviant adult populations presupposes that the anomalies in question are unassociated with special mortality risks; furthermore, the two populations do not differ significantly by a number of variables of a socioeconomic, medical or biologic nature.[19] The argument is compelling that the frequencies obtained in newborn surveys of XXY, XXX and XYY will not satisfy our epidemiologic requirements, and we shall need to examine random population groups of other ages.

One such study in progress is a collaborative one that plans to examine 11,000 children aged 8 and 9 years. Of the 1,800 surveyed thus far, three XYY males have been found, and no XXY males or XXX females.[20] Another study of 1,715 school boys failed to reveal a single XYY individual.[21] Despite the considerable investments of the investigators, the relatively small population size in both studies raises serious doubt as to the validity of the frequency estimates they will generate.

Should we obtain data on the sex chromosome anomalies by chromosomal surveys, or should sex-chromatin methods of population screening be encouraged?

Sex-chromatin studies of nondividing cells make use of the cytologic recognition of inactivated X chromosomes in stained whole-cell preparations. They were used effectively in screening both newborn as well as special populations even before methods were available to study human chromosomes. The accuracy in recognizing XXY males and XXX females by this technic has been validated.[22] Table 3 compares the incidence of sex chromosome aneuploidy estimated by newborn sex chromosome with similar estimates by sex-chromatin surveys.

There are no significant differences between the frequencies of X chromosome aneuploidy detected by chromatin and chromosome surveys even though there are certain apparent discrepancies, especially with regard to XXX frequencies, that deserve further evaluation. The ease with which large numbers can be screened by the chromatin technics argues for their use in determining the prevalence of sex chromosome aneuploidy in different age groups. Quinacrine staining of interphase cells has been described as an effective method of screening populations for abnormalities of the Y chromosome.[23,24] Presumably this procedure can be applied to screening for XYY males with the same effectiveness that sex-chromatin methods have been used in screening for XXY males and XXX females. Careful validation of this approach to XYY screening will be needed before applying it to mass surveys.[25]

Table 3. Frequency of Sex Chromosome Aneuploidy: Comparison of Chromosome and Chromatin Surveys of Newborns

	Chromosomes	*No. Surveyed*	*Chromatin*	*No. Surveyed*
Males:				
XXY	1.2/1,000	11,039	1.10/1,000	72,538
XX	0.1/1,000		0.60/1,000	
Females:				
XXX	1.1/1,000	5,608	0.58/1,000	68,924
XO	0.2/1,000		0.10/1,000	

Robinson et al are applying the sex-chromatin technic to newborn screening.[26] This approach permits the study of large numbers of consecutive newborns by modest-sized laboratories, and therefore allows for the accumulation of considerably more data on sex chromosome aneuploidy than would screening procedures that employ chromosome analysis. It has already been shown that seasonal and random fluctuations in the frequency of sex chromosome aneuploidy can result in gross errors of incidence estimation when small samples are used; eg in Robinson's survey consecutive sequences of 5,000 newborn infants have been observed with no X chromosome aneuploidy.[22] It would thus appear from preliminary estimates of the frequency of sex chromosome aneuploidy that sample sizes of 50,000 to 100,000 may be needed to obtain valid epidemiologic information.

To restate the problem: There are three sex chromosome aneuploidies (XXY, XXX, XYY) that occur with appreciable frequency in chromosome surveys of newborn populations. It is important to refine these data not only for the newborn population, but also for other age groups in order to compare, with confidence, normal populations with deviant ones. Chromatin surveys appear to provide comparable data to the chromosome surveys, and the use of chromatin methods allows for the more efficient acquisition of large amounts of data.

The critical question, however, is why acquisition of these kinds of data on the occurrence of these three sex chromosome aneuploidies is warranted. This question can be better answered after looking individually at these three conditions.

XXX

There is considerable uncertainty as to the phenotypic expression of the triple-X chromosome constitution. The tentative conclusions drawn from reviewing the recorded observations of XXX children and adults are that the majority of these individuals have a normal reproductive system, and an uncertain proportion have congenital defects of a physical nature.[27] The latter characteristic may well be influenced by the method of ascertaining the described individuals. There is considerable evidence from sex-chromatin surveys that there is a higher rate of triple-X females in institutions for the mentally retarded than in newborn populations.[20,27] There has been little or no special attention paid to this entity by disciplines interested in problems of learning, and there is no evidence that XXX individuals have special adaptation problems other than those related to their learning disability.

XYY

The XYY dilemma has been thoroughly aired in both the popular and scientific press. There is no doubt that the frequency of males with an XYY complement is greater in certain types of security hospitals or prisons than in the newborn population.[6] Evidence to date suggests that an extra Y chromosome does not markedly affect intelligence, but may in an undefined way influence social behavior.[20] As with the XXX data, appropriate control populations have not been studied; so prevalences in special populations have been compared principally with those obtained in surveys of newborn infants.

An excellent synthesis has been made by Hook[28] of the current status of information about the significance of an XYY genotype: "Discovery of an extra sex chromosome (ie Y chromosome) in a male hardly predicts antisocial behavior with the confidence, for instance, that the observation of trisomy 21 predicts mental retardation." He further concludes that "Telling the parents of the diagnosis and possible prognosis is likely to induce more difficulties for both child and family than not informing them, particularly since the precise behavioral risks are uncertain and there are no therapeutic preventive measures known at present that are specific for an individual with the XYY genotype."

XXY

The XXY phenotype in contrast to both the XXX and XYY is nearly always associated with significant abnormalities of gonadal function, both in terms of reproductive capacity and hormonal homeostasis (the so-called Klinefelter syndrome). Surveys of populations of males with compromised mental function have established with reasonable confidence that the XXY individual is likely to be found in institutions for the moderately retarded (IQ around 50), more so than in those for the severely retarded. The severely retarded individual is more likely to be identified and sequestered by society than the deviant who is closer to the population norm.

Therefore, it is likely that most XXY individuals, even with intellectual limitations, exist outside of institutions.

Since XXY males are frequently ascertained because of physical reasons (small testes, gynecomastia, infertility), it is reasonable to examine the clinical information on the behavioral characteristics of such individuals.[29] Comparison of hypogonadal males who are XY with those who are XXY reveals that the latter group more frequently demonstrates lower school performance, poorer relations with parents or sibs, or a history of mental illness.[20] In one group of 50 Klinefelter patients, mental deficiency was infrequent, while severe psychiatric disorders occurred in one third and was of clinical significance in another third.[30]

There is compelling evidence that hormonal aberrations may well play a major role in the social maladjustment of many XXY males. Research in the metabolism of testicular hormones in man has advanced our understanding of androgen function in both normal and XXY males.[31,32] The role of androgen has in recent years become a major interest of behavioral scientists. There have been encouraging preliminary reports of favorable responses of XXY children appropriately treated with androgens.[33,34]

Hook has argued that the diagnosis of XXY, like XYY, is of no benefit to the affected individual and his parents because of our ignorance of its phenotypic spectrum and our inability to offer therapeutic possibilities. From our viewpoint, however, it would appear that the XXY situation is different from that of either XYY or XXX. Perhaps this difference of opinion is more apparent than real, since the outcome of clinical investigations that involve therapeutic approaches to XXY persons is not yet available. Nonetheless, can the medical profession and society continue to neglect this sizable group of patients who suffer significant degrees of social maladjustment, or should they be made aware of their diagnosis and be invited to participate in investigations of potential therapeutic benefit to them?

What should be our future goals and our method of approaching sex chromosome aneuploidy in human populations?

The problem of the XXY male should be separated from those of the XYY male and XXX female. Information already available about the XXY individual would seem to justify a major effort by clinical investigators, and therefore the recruitment of subjects should be done by established medical research agencies. Large population groups need to be surveyed by sex-chromatin methods to identify significant numbers of XXY subjects in childhood. There is no special justification for testing newborns for this purpose. What is the appropriate age group can be debated; it might be age 6 years (when entering the educational process) or 10 (when the early signs of gonadal maturation, at least by laboratory criteria, are usually in evidence), or it might be more broadly defined to include entire school populations. Programs of study and therapeutic experimentation must be implemented by the combined resources of scientists concerned with learning and behavior and those who deal with hormonal regulation and metabolism.

The study population should be enlisted by established voluntary consent procedures, at least for the investigations of identified XXY subjects, almost certain to involve trials with therapeutic agents. Claims of beneficial effects of therapies will need scientific validation, and will require experiments with control (placebo-treated) groups.

Should voluntary procedures be insisted upon for the identification of XXY individuals in these study populations?

Legislation might be enacted that would require the sex-chromatin screening of males to diagnose XXY individuals. The age of the study population might be specified, just as the age that a state requires children to enter into compulsory education. There is ample precedent for this in legislation, existing in nearly all of the states of the United States, that requires the testing of all newborn infants for phenylketonuria. (See also the review by Green and Capron in this series.) Most such laws do not require study and treatment, only screening for the disease.

Certainly, such compulsory diagnosis of XXY males should come only after the appropriate legislative bodies have been convinced of the wisdom of establishing this type of mass survey for the purpose of identifying a research population – clearly a novel, but perhaps not unreasonable, alliance between medical science and the political process. The adoption of such a process would presumably occur after a legislature has been convinced that special education methods, preventive mental health technics and hormonal therapies would result in sufficient benefit to the population of XXY individuals, estimated to constitute 0.1%-0.2% of males. The individuals concerned, if experimental therapies were indeed beneficial, could become more productive and happier members of society, and there would be a corresponding reduction in the demands on publicly supported custodial institutions that include security hospitals and prisons.

Having suggested the possibility of a compulsory screening program for XXY males and having invoked the precedent of PKU screening laws, one is chastened by a statement that appeared in *The New York Times*: "Nowadays when people get an idea about a thing, they become enthusiastic and rush to pass laws, before they know what they are doing." This comment appeared in 1914 and was authored by C. B. Davenport.[35]

Realistically, and perhaps more properly, population surveys to identify XXY children can be done through voluntary programs, and the consenting parents would be informed in advance of the investigative protocols planned for identified individuals.

XYY and XXX

The objectives in detecting XYY and XXX females are distinct from those described for XXY males. Better estimates of prevalences in random populations during the first 20 years of life, and the phenotypes of these chromosomally abnormal states in children, adolescents and young adults would be desirable. *Since there is no basis for implying that such screening leads to therapeutic benefit to individuals or provides useful information to parents, these studies should not be promoted to the public as medical research.* The use of physicians and hospital settings to obtain population genetic data, when there is no health benefit for the individuals concerned, must be questioned. Newborn chromosome surveys, by definition, are medically oriented studies. The public does not have the sophistication to make the distinction, in providing consent for research, between volunteering for procedures that are of no health value to them or their families and for procedures which have therapeutic content, when they are solicited in a medical environment.

Although the only obvious alternative setting for acquiring the large random populations needed is in the schools, we would argue that informed consent here is less coercive than in medical facilities.

If male and female populations are to be screened for XYY or XXX chromosomal constitutions, chromatin technics should be used, since these methods make it feasible to test the large populations required for obtaining significant data. Furthermore, there would need to be absolute guarantees of anonymity to the volunteering subjects. Should follow-up studies of any type, including confirmatory chromosome studies, be planned, the subjects would need to be so informed in advance. Any planned follow-up would perforce prohibit anonymous sampling and probably jeopardize the rate of voluntary participation. Objection to such anonymous studies might be raised, because phenotype data would not be available to correlate with the chromatin findings. A possible way of meeting this objection would be to use coded questionnaires to record the behavioral traits of the subjects. Questionnaires could be completed by a school official when the specimens for sex chromatin are obtained. At no time would the volunteer's name appear on either the sample slide or questionnaire, and coded slides and questionnaires could be matched in order to correlate chromatin and phenotype data. It must be accepted that the use of anonymity-assuring technics will reduce the information yield.

If investigators plan to perform behavioral studies on either abnormal or control subjects who volunteer to be screened for XYY or XXX, this should be part of the information provided at the time consent is obtained. The subjects who volunteer for a survey under such conditions could be remarkably different from those who agree to participate in a study that guarantees anonymity and assures in advance that there will not be follow-up studies.

Conclusion

From an examination of current information about the cytogenetics of human populations it would appear that more novel data-gathering approaches may be needed to advance our understanding of the XXY, XXX and XYY sex chromosome aneuploidies.

Answers to questions now being asked about XYY and XXX individuals can be expected to provide insights in the areas of learning and behavior, but not health – at least as health is construed by the public. Therefore, studies to identify and investigate these two genetic abnormalities should not be disguised by a medical research environment. Major social issues which must be faced to accomplish research goals concerning these anomalies involve the classic ones of informed consent and guarantees of nondisclosure and confidentiality.

Prevalence data for ages other than the newborn are badly needed by behavioral scientists and cytogeneticists, and population sizes of 50,000 to 100,000 may be required to acquire reliable estimates. Although absolute guarantees of nondisclosure should always be provided in such surveys, it is likely that more accurate prevalence data can be acquired by a program that assures the anonymity of the participants.

Definition of XYY and XXX phenotypes by the process of identifying individuals in newborn surveys and studying them from birth until social maturity is too slow to satisfy society's impatience for this information. Alternatively, these chromosome aberrations can be characterized longitudinally by finding cases through mass surveys of different age groups and piecing together these vertically derived data. Chromatin technics are the most efficient methods of acquiring the necessary population samples.

As currently perceived, there are intrinsic differences between the biomedical significance of the XYY and XXX genotypes on the one hand and that of the XXY on the other. The care and investigation of XXY individuals, who are generally recognized to have disorders of body and mind, are proper medical concerns. Although there is currently no basis for promoting the study of XYY and XXX by legislative fiat, there exists the question (perhaps raised out of devilment) of whether society can or should require the identification of its XXY members, if it believes that the proposed therapeutic investigations may benefit these individuals. Superficially at least, there is little or no substantial difference between legislating XXY screening and the existing PKU screening laws. Society appears to look upon the latter program, which is applied to newborn infants, as a benevolence of the state, not an abridgment of individual choice. Or is the newborn a special class of citizen distinct from the XXY male, who might best be screened for at age 6, 10 or older?

The dilemmas are profound, yet the stage has now been reached in the acquisition of knowledge about the chromosomes of human populations when geneticists and society should consider together how best to obtain and apply such information.

References

1. Rutovitz, D., Cameron, J., Farrow, A. S. J. et al: Instrumentation and organization for chromosome measurement and karyotype analysis. *Pfizer Med. Mono. (Human Population Cytogenetics), 5*:282, 1969.
2. Wald, N., Ranshaw, R. W., Herron, J. M. and Castle, J. G.: Progress on an automatic system for cytogenetic analysis. *Pfizer Med. Mono. (Human Population Cytogenetics), 5*:264, 1969.
3. Wright, S. W., Crandall, B. F. and Boyer, L. (eds.): *Perspectives in Cytogenetics.* Springfield:Charles C Thomas, 1972, p. 309.
4. Nowell, P. C. and Hungerford, D. A.: Chromosome studies on normal and leukemic human leukocytes. *J. Nat. Cancer Inst., 25*:85, 1962.
5. Buckton, K. E., Jacobs, P. A., Court-Brown, W. M. and Doll, R.: A study of the chromosome damage persisting after x-ray therapy for ankylosing spondylitis. *Lancet, 2*:676, 1962.
6. Smith, P. G. and Jacobs, P. A.: Incidence studies of constitutional chromosome abnormalities in the post-natal population. *Pfizer Med. Mono. (Human Population Cytogenetics), 5*:160, 1970.
7. Court-Brown, W. M., Buckton, K. E., Jacobs, P. A. et al: *Chromosome Studies on Adults.* Eugenics Lab. Mem. No. 42, Galton Lab., University College, London. London:Cambridge University Press, 1966.
8. Jacobs, P. A., Brunton, M., Melville, M. M. et al: Aggressive behaviour, mental subnormality and the XYY male. *Nature (London), 208*:1351, 1965.

9. Jacobs, P. A., Price, W. H., Court-Brown, W. M. et al: Chromosome studies on men in a maximum security hospital. *Ann. Hum. Genet., 31*:339, 1968.
10. Casey, M. D., Blank, C. E., Street, D. R. K. et al: YY chromosomes and antisocial behaviour. *Lancet, 2*:859, 1966.
11. Court-Brown, W. M.: Males with an XYY sex chromosome complement. *J. Med. Genet., 5*:341, 1968.
12. Craig-Holmes, A. P., Moore, F. B. and Shaw, M. W.: Polymorphism of human C-band heterochromatin I. Frequency of variants. *Amer. J. Hum. Genet., 25*:181, 1973.
13. Lubs, H., Patel, S., Kimberling, W. et al: Correlations between low I.Q., race and variations in Q and C banding. *Amer. J. Hum. Genet., 25*:47a, 1973.
14. Eller, E., Frankenburg, W., Puck, M. and Robinson, A.: Prognosis in newborn infants with X-chromosomal abnormalities. *Pediatrics, 47*:681, 1971.
15. de la Chapelle, A.: Nature and origin of males with XX sex chromosomes. *Amer. J. Hum. Genet., 24*:71, 1972.
16. Court-Brown, W. M. and Smith, P. G.: Human population cytogenetics. *Brit. Med. Bull., 25*:74, 1969.
17. Court-Brown, W. M.: Sex chromosome aneuploidy. *Int. Rev. Exp. Path.*, 7:31, 1969.
18. *Report on the XYY Chromosomal Abnormality,* bulletin 2103. U. S. Public Health Service, National Institutes of Mental Health, 1970.
19. Kessler, S. and Moos, R. H.: Behavioral aspects of chromosomal disorders. *Ann. Rev. Med., 24*:89, 1973.
20. Patil, S., Lubs, H., Kimberling, W. et al: Chromosome abnormalities in 7 and 8 year old children. *Amer. J. Hum. Genet., 25*:58a, 1973.
21. Borgaonkar, D. S.: Chromosome survey of Maryland boys. *Amer. J. Hum. Genet., 24*:13a, 1972.
22. Wright, S. W., Crandall, B. F. and Boyer, L. (eds.): *Perspectives in Cytogenetics.* Springfield:Charles C Thomas, 1972, p. 297.
23. Greensher, A., Gersh, R., Peakman, D. and Robinson, A.: Screening of newborn infants for abnormalities of the Y chromosome. *J. Pediat., 79*:305, 1971.
24. Dorus, E. B., Dorus, W. and Telfer, M. A.: Prevalence and personality characteristics of 47,XYY males in a sample of non-institutionalized males. *Amer. J. Hum. Genet., 25*:24a, 1973.
25. Hsu, L. Y. F., Dubin, E. C., Kerenyi, T. and Hirschorn, K.: Results and pitfalls in prenatal cytogenetic diagnosis. *J. Med. Genet., 10*:112, 1973.
26. Robinson, A., Goad, W. B., Puck, T. T. and Harris, J. S.: Studies on chromosomal nondisjunction in man III. *Amer. J. Hum. Genet., 21*:466, 1969.
27. Barr, M. L., Sergovich, F. R., Carr, D. H. and Shaver, E. L.: The triple-X female: An appraisal based on a study of 12 cases and a review of the literature. *Canad. Med. Ass. J., 101*:247-258, 1969.
28. Hook, E. B.: Behavioral implications of the human XYY genotype. *Science, 179*:139, 1973.
29. Kaplan, N. M. and Norfleet, R. G.: Hypogonadism in young men (with emphasis on Klinefelter's syndrome). *Ann. Int. Med., 54*:461-481, 1961.
30. Becker, K. L., Hoffman, D. L., Albert, A. et al: Klinefelter's syndrome. *Arch. Int. Med., 118*:314, 1966.
31. Lipsett, M. B., Davis, T. E., Wilson, H. and Canfield, C. J.: Testosterone

production in chromatin-positive Klinefelter's syndrome. *J. Clin. Endocrinol. Metab., 25*:1027, 1965.
32. Stewart-Bentley, M. and Horton, R.: Leydig function in Klinefelter's syndrome. *Metabolism, 22*:875, 1973.
33. Myhre, S. A., Ruvalcaba, R. H. A., Johnson, H. R. et al: The effects of testosterone treatment in Klinefelter's syndrome. *J. Pediat., 76*:267, 1970.
34. Caldwell, P. D. and Smith, D. W.: The XXY (Klinefelter's) syndrome in childhood: Detection and treatment. *J. Pediat., 80*:250, 1972.
35. Haller, M. H.: In *Eugenics.* New Brunswick:Rutgers University Press, 1963, p. 132.

Informed Consent in Genetic Screening Programs

**John Fletcher, Th.D., Richard O. Roblin, Ph.D.
and Tabitha M. Powledge, M.S.**

In 1972, the Research Group on ethical, social and legal issues in genetic counseling and genetic engineering of the Institute of Society, Ethics and the Life Sciences published an article concerning ethical and social issues in screening for genetic disease.[1] The article addressed a number of ethical problems in the context of an anticipated rapid rise in large-scale screening programs to detect and counsel heterozygous carriers. Among those problems was the question of obtaining an informed consent from those entering a screening program. The article stated:

> Screening should be conducted only with the informed consent of those tested or of the parents or legal representatives of minors . . . In addition to obtaining signed consent documents, it is the program director's obligation to assure that knowledgeable consent is obtained from all those screened, to design and implement informational procedures, and to review the consent procedure for its effectiveness.

The concept of informed consent put forward by the research group, which contained a number of geneticists involved with screening programs, was based on the requirement in medical research that a physician-investigator inform a patient or his representative of the purpose, risks and benefits of an investigative procedure, and then obtain consent from the patient. Because this understanding of the consent requirement was a part of its deliberations, the group recommended the guidelines on protection of human subjects, available from the Department of Health, Education and Welfare, as "a useful model for formulating such consent procedures."[1]

John Fletcher, Th.D., *Director, Interfaith Metropolitan Theological Education, Inc., Washington, D. C.;* Richard O. Roblin, Ph.D., *Assistant Professor, Harvard Medical School, Infectious Disease Unit, Massachusetts General Hospital, Boston; and* Tabitha M. Powledge, M.S., *Research Associate for Genetics, Institute of Society, Ethics and the Life Sciences, Hastings-on-Hudson, N. Y.*

The article prompted a number of questions about the feasibility of obtaining person-to-person informed consent in large-scale genetic screening programs. Among the questioners was Robert Q. Marston, then director of the National Institutes of Health:

> The participle "informed" can have many meanings. Quite clearly, each participant in a screening program cannot be educated to the level of a professional geneticist; yet, even the professional geneticist's information is obviously limited. The question of how informed you anticipate the screenee to be is an open-ended one.[2]

Such questions, and the realization that geneticists in the group were practicing, in their own screening programs, a standard far short of the one expressed in the statement, led the authors to wonder if the research group's informed consent requirement had been so strict as to be unattainable in practice. We therefore carried out a preliminary study designed to determine the operational concepts of informed consent held by directors of several genetic screening programs. The evidence of practice is compared here with the informed consent standard contained in the original article. Discussion of the results of interviews with program directors follows, and we conclude with some suggestions for obtaining prior informed consent in genetic screening programs.

Our working hypothesis for the interviews was that program directors would reject direct applicability of the informed consent requirement to genetic screening, and that they would argue that such screening was not different from other public health screening programs in which there is currently no informed consent requirement. We thought they would say the fact that a person presents himself for screening constitutes his implied consent to the procedures.

Six interviews were conducted with program directors in four cities in the eastern United States. These program directors were associated with community-based, hospital-based or research center-based screening programs for the carrier state of two recessive conditions, Tay-Sachs disease and sickle cell anemia. Answers to a standardized set of questions were unexpectedly diverse and do not lend themselves to tabular presentation, so we shall discuss some of the questions and the range of responses separately.

How do you understand the meaning or force of consent in genetic screening?

There was considerable divergence of opinion among the six program directors on this question. Positions ranged from the view that appearance of the screenee at the test site constituted implied consent (Screeners A and E) to the view that written consent forms were desirable (Screener F). As an example of the implied consent position, one program director stated:

> My attitude is that if people make an appointment and come in voluntarily, that constitutes consent. They get information. At any point they wish they could decide not to take the test, and some don't. From a practical standpoint, the members of the staff feel that the risks are minimal anyway. Going through rigid informed consent procedures might get in the way, and we do not want to keep people from the test. (Screener A)

At the other end of the spectrum, another program director responded:

> Well, I certainly think it means a written consent. I don't think it means a verbal consent. That's one rather simple thing. (Screener F)

Our survey of consent practices revealed that two programs required some form of written consent for the blood test (Screeners B and F), one program was in the process of developing a written consent form (Screener C), one program regarded completion of a prescreening questionnaire as tantamount to implied consent (Screener D), and two programs used no formal consent procedures (although one of the last two did require written consent from parents or guardians of minors. (Screeners A and E)

Do the HEW human experimentation guidelines apply to genetic screening programs?

All six program directors responded that they did *not* think so. Five of them stated that voluntary screening programs were a public health service, not a research project, and thus human experimentation guidelines did not apply. As one program director put it:

> Screening is a well-established chapter in public medicine. Its earlier forms were screening for TB, glaucoma, heart disease, diabetes and hypertension. There are all sorts of side effects of medical screening, but people are not told about them. (Screener A)

However, two program directors (Screeners E and F) indicated that if a screening program incorporated additional research components, such as in-depth attitude studies, then the HEW human experimentation guidelines should become applicable. In addition, one program director somewhat qualified his general position that the HEW guidelines did not apply:

I think it may be wiser for the persons who are involved in this to look at it from the point of view that it has the potential for experimentation, even though this (experimentation) may not be the objective of the individual (screener). But it has that potential, and therefore should be treated with the kind of respect that experimentation requires . . . Whether or not we are actually in experimentation in screening I am not quite certain that I can answer . . . what we do is not for the immediate benefit of the patient; it is for information which the screenee can use in an informed way at some subsequent time . . . Where I think the whole problem is . . . is that there is no trust, and this is where the whole issue has reared its head. There has been a chasm created between the person performing the tests and the recipient . . . Things have occurred over the course of time which have provoked a warranted sense of concern that things that have been done have not been in the best interest of the person who has been screened . . . Until we find the way to restore confidence and trust, we will be splitting more and more hairs. (Screener F)

What are the risks involved in genetic screening programs?

All program directors agreed that the risk involved in taking the blood sample for testing was negligible, but that there were elements of sociopsychologic risk that had to be considered. Among the comments:

"There is a very minimal risk from taking blood. The main risks are economic, to privacy, and a risk of stigmatization. I know of one person who lost his job because he was found to be a carrier. We do not discuss these risks with the screenees. There is a risk in losing your job if you are found to be a sickle cell carrier and you are an airline pilot." (Screener A)

"The risk is psychological, like a person may have false knowledge about being a carrier and worry a lot; another person may not be able to handle the information and distort it. There is also a social risk, which results from the public's ignorance about genetics, which may result in a certain amount of stigmatization." (Screener B)

"Stigmatization . . . psychological consequences . . . anxiety." (Screener C)

"We can't currently evaluate the impact on the individual found to be a carrier." (Screener E)

"These are the risks that I can see: one, from the point of view of the patient, is the unnecessary, anxiety-provoking, stigmatizing thing; the second being the risk of misinformation, either because of technique or bookkeeping; and thirdly, the very small medical element of risk involved in the actual procedures." (Screener F)

Taken together, the comments indicate that these six program directors regarded possible adverse social and psychologic reactions as the major risks to the screenee. However, since there is as yet little reliable information about the frequency of such adverse reactions, the program directors opposed discussing these possible risks with screenees before testing.

What is it that you would like each screenee to know?

There was some ambiguity in this question, since it was not specified whether the screenee should know this information *before* or *after* screening. However, the following pieces of information were said to be desirable by one or more program directors:

1. The incurability of the disease.
2. The influence on reproductive life.
3. The involvement of personal privacy.
4. An understanding of the program and its purposes.
5. How the information will be used.
6. The confidentiality of the information.
7. The odds of having an affected child.
8. The nature of the disease.
9. The difference between a carrier and a homozygote.
10. How the condition might affect the patient, his or her offspring and subsequent generations.
11. How the knowledge might influence a screenee's choice of mate.
12. Better knowledge about genetic abnormalities in general.

We found that no single concern was mentioned by all – or even most – screening program directors.

Other Relevant Comments

One director (of Program B) was aware that his educational material did not mention consent issues and what he would like the screenee to know, but another supervisor of that program was not aware whether the material mentioned the consent issue at all. They thought that it would be possible to add a page dealing with consent questions to the current questionnaire. All directors indicated a willingness to experiment with different consent procedures to assure quality informed consent. Some felt the chief problem was lack of personnel and funds. Half of the program directors expressed concern that too much information given to potential screenees might frighten them out of being tested. (Screeners A, C and F)

Conclusions and Recommendations

The fact that two out of six of the program directors interviewed said they require written informed consent prior to screening disproves our original hypothesis that program directors reject the applicability of a formal consent procedure to genetic screening. One program director stated his needs in the following way:

> I want guidelines . . . I reject the idea that genetic screening is a special case which exempts it from the norm of informed consent . . . I would not let the program directors out from under. They will tend to set up shoddy programs if you do. (Screener B)

An alternative hypothesis, drawn from the pluralistic set of informed consent practices we discovered in our interviews, is that there is some agreement about the theoretic desirability of obtaining prior informed consent in genetic screening programs. There is, however, little agreement about what the screenee should know before being tested, nor about how quality informed consent can be obtained from the large numbers of people who will be tested in mass genetic screening programs.

Being identified as a carrier of a recessive genetic disease is a new and undefined role, and the genetic screener is responsible for initiating the screenee into this new role. Accordingly, the screener also bears a responsibility for the possibly disruptive consequences of informing screenees that they are carriers, at least until our society has a chance to adjust to the meaning of this new knowledge, and to minimize possible discrimination, stigmatization and feelings of inadequacy resulting from it. We believe it is important for genetic screening programs to determine the frequency and severity of adverse social and psychologic reactions to the testing process by appropriate postscreening follow-up studies. Whether or not such evaluations are carried out depends, in large measure, upon the availability of funds. Recent experience suggests that it may be easier to obtain money for genetic screening *per se* than for evaluation of the possible adverse side effects of screening. We urge the National Institutes of Health to give the highest funding priority to genetic screening proposals which include a built-in evaluation of social and psychologic reactions to screening.

Incorporation of procedures which aim at obtaining informed consent in genetic screening programs would serve several functions. First, requiring understanding of the procedures, goals, risks and benefits of the genetic screening program *prior* to the testing process would maximize the freedom of individual prospective screenees to make informed choices about whether they want this information about their genotypes. It would thus minimize any coercive elements inherent in the recruitment aspects of mass genetic screening programs. In addition, obtaining prior informed consent could enhance the vital public education component of genetic screening by providing program directors with a way of assessing the effectiveness of their prescreening informational materials.

Thus, we believe that the original statement of the Research Group should not be softened in its intent. From our interviews with the program directors, it appears that barriers to obtaining prior informed consent lie in lack of funds, personnel and imagination to approach the informed consent ideal in large-scale screening programs. We therefore favor the following amplification of the original statement on informed consent by the genetics research group:

> This statement of obligation is made with awareness of the difficulties of direct person-to-person application of informed consent procedures, since screening usually involves working with large groups. As a practical approach to the ideal of individualized person-to-person informed consent, we suggest the use of an informed consent questionnaire [such as the one below], which is adaptable to the purposes of individual screening programs. This consent sheet of questions could be used singly or added to the prescreening informational materials, if any are used in the program. In addition, we recommend that the program director or his designee review the answers to the informed consent questionnaire *before* each individual is tested, in order to complete the education of potential screenees who remain confused about important aspects of the genetic screening program.
>
> We argue that heterozygote screening is a new and not-yet-evaluated medical procedure, with unknown sociopsychologic risks, and should therefore be treated as a research procedure as far as consent is concerned.

Sample Informed Consent Questionnaire

(The program should fill in the blanks to make this form fit its procedure. This list of questions is intended to be suggestive rather than exhaustive.)

Because this genetic screening is voluntary, we want you to be as well-informed as possible. If you can answer "YES" to each statement below, and give your consent to be screened, please sign the sheet and we will proceed with the test. If you are not certain about any item here, please check "NO" and a staff member will try to make it clearer.

1. I have read the informational material __(title)__ about ___(name of disease)___ provided by this program. ___ YES ___ NO

2. I understand that the purpose of this program is to ___(program fills in)___ ___ YES ___ NO

3. I understand that if I am found to be a carrier of the __(disease)__ gene, I will be offered further consultation and counseling. ___ YES ___ NO

4. I understand that the odds I am a carrier of _(disease)_ are about one in _(heterozygote frequency in this population)_

   ___ ___
   YES NO

5. I understand that a positive result of the test may affect my decisions about having children.

   ___ ___
   YES NO

6. I understand that all information derived from this test is confidential and will not be released to any party without my consent

   ___ ___
   YES NO

Because I consider myself informed on these questions, I voluntarily give my consent for a blood test to be screened for carrier status in _(disease)_

__________ DATE

__________ SIGNATURE

References

1. Genetics Research Group: Ethical and social issues in screening for genetic disease. *N. Eng. J. Med., 286*:1129, 1972.
2. Marston, R. Q.: Written communication to M. Lappé, 1972.

Sociologic Studies in Human Genetics

I. Compliance Factors in a Voluntary Heterozygote Screening Program

**Michael M. Kaback, M.D., Marshall H. Becker, Ph.D.
and M. Virginia Ruth, M.S.N.**

Introduction and Background

It is believed that genetic counseling has been an effective instrument in the prevention of genetic disease. For example, when a defined genetic condition is detected in an individual, counseling of the parents and close relatives is often associated with a reduction in further occurrences of the disorder in that family. After the family is informed of the nature and prognosis of the disease in question and of the statistical probability for recurrence in future offspring, many families choose to avoid further reproduction.[1] This is particularly the case in families where the condition is severe and untreatable and in which a substantial risk for recurrence of the disease is known (ie Tay-Sachs disease, cystic fibrosis, sickle cell anemia, etc.).[2] The significant risk of additional affected offspring and, perhaps more important, the substantial emotional or financial burden which such diseases often impart have been reported to be sufficient to result in a voluntary cessation of further reproduction.[3] Unfortunately, the burden and associated guilt felt by parents who have had a child with an untreatable, inherited condition frequently has led to family disruption and lifelong stigmatization of the remaining healthy individuals.

These studies were supported by The John F. Kennedy Institute, Tay-Sachs Disease Fund, Aaron and Lillian Strauss Foundation, Maryland State Department of Health and Mental Hygiene, The National Foundation-March of Dimes, The California Community Foundation, The National Capitol Tay-Sachs Association and contributions from other organizations and individuals.

Michael M. Kaback, M.D., *Associate Chief, Division of Medical Genetics, Departments of Pediatrics and Medicine, UCLA School of Medicine-Harbor General Hospital, Torrance;* Marshall H. Becker, Ph.D. *and* M. Virginia Ruth, M.S.N., *School of Public Health, The Johns Hopkins University, Baltimore, Md.*

The recent development of technics for the accurate intrauterine diagnosis of certain genetic diseases in the fetus during early pregnancy, plus the changing social and legal attitudes toward abortion, has significantly altered the situation described above and has added a new parameter to the scope of genetic counseling. Now, couples need no longer fear the recurrence of specific genetic diseases in their offspring. If, through amniocentesis and amniotic fluid cell analysis, the disorder can be detected in the fetus in early pregnancy, families who in the past might have been unwilling to risk reproduction can now be availed a mechanism by which they can have further children without fear of the disease. This implies, of course, that such families would elect to monitor their pregnancies with amniocentesis and to terminate those pregnancies in which an affected fetus is identified. Since the recurrence risk for genetic disease is rarely greater than 25% (and most often is substantially less), at-risk families can now, with confidence, take the more-than-likely opportunity to have unaffected offspring.

This dramatically alters the mechanism by which genetic disease is prevented. In the past genetic disease prevention was achieved through limitation of further reproduction in these families. Now at-risk couples can reproduce and, at the same time, selectively prevent further cases of the disorder in question, if the new alternative is acceptable to them.

Another important and related advance in the preventive control of genetic disease is the development of simple, accurate and relatively inexpensive technics for the identification of healthy individuals who are heterozygous for specific recessive genes (carriers). The capability to detect recessive disease carriers provides an important new tool for the potential control of many human genetic diseases. In families in which recessive disorders have been identified, carrier detection may greatly improve the accuracy of genetic counseling for unaffected relatives. In a larger sense, carrier identification for genes which have a particular predilection for a defined subpopulation may allow the identification of individuals or couples at risk for such conditions in their offspring, even before an index case has occurred.

Carrier Detection And Disease Prevention

Heterozygote identification methods have been described for a number of X-linked and autosomal recessive conditions.[4,5] In only a few, however, (ie sickle cell anemia, Tay-Sachs disease and thalassemia) are the characteristics of the disorder such, and are the methods for carrier detection sufficiently accurate, simple and inexpensive, to warrant consideration for populational screening at this time. Much more than the availability of a test method must be considered before it is decided to screen substantial populations for deleterious recessive genes. What are the goals of such an effort? Who, when and how are people to be screened? What alternatives will be available for individuals or couples found to carry such genes? It is essential that these and several other issues be critically evaluated before massive populational screening is initiated.

If effective control of disease through prevention is to be the goal of a carrier screening program, then several approaches could be considered. For autosomal recessive conditions in which no treatment or preventive method is available, carrier screening might be conducted prior to marriage. Identified carriers could than be counseled concerning the implications of their carrier status. A carrier identified premaritally could be advised of the risk he or she would incur for genetic disease in his offspring if he reproduced with another individual carrying the same recessive gene. Unquestionably, *if* counseling could be effective in this situation, and *if* such information could be used by identified carriers without causing major psychologic or social difficulties for them, then genetic disease prevention would be achieved. It must be recognized, however, that disease prevention is achieved in this way by an implicit restriction on the mate selection choices of the individual. In addition, the potential for psychologic and social stigmatization of the "carriers" in their interactions with peers might be considerable. When and how the matter of heterozygosity would be introduced and discussed among young dating individuals is a matter of conjecture, but nonetheless, concern. On the other hand, carrier detection for such a condition, at or after the time of marriage, might reveal a couple's state of genetic risk after important and deep commitments have already been made. Such a discovery at that time could result in extraordinary difficulties for the couple.

Where the heterozygous condition for a given disorder can be identified, *and where prenatal diagnosis of the condition is possible,* the situation becomes considerably different. Carrier detection programs here might be directed *primarily* to young married couples. Through screening, at-risk couples (in which both husband and wife are heterozygotes) could be identified and then counseled as to their alternatives, including prenatal diagnosis. This would permit the delineation of at-risk couples before the disease has occurred and provide an alternative by which they could still reproduce without fear of the disease in question. In this way, carrier detection neither imposes limitations on mate selection nor on the reproductive aspirations of those individuals and couples who accept this method.

Tay-Sachs Disease: The Model

Tay-Sachs disease (TSD) is the first recessive condition in which a prospective approach to disease prevention has been applied.[6] Three considerations, unique to this condition, provide the rationale for this effort:

1. The disease occurs in a defined population, thereby making effective screening feasible. TSD occurs 100 times more frequently in Jewish infants of Eastern and central European ancestry (Ashkenazi Jews). The heterozygote frequency is estimated to be about 1 in 30 in this group and about 1 in 300 among non-Jews. About 1 in 900 Jewish couples, therefore, would be expected to be at risk for TSD in their offspring.[7]
2. Activity of the lysosomal isoenzyme hexosaminidase A (Hex A), is significantly reduced in the tissues, blood cells and body fluids of individuals heterozygous for this recessive gene, compared with that in noncarriers.[8]
3. An accurate method for the prenatal detection of TSD exists.[9,10] Activity of Hex A is totally deficient in the amniotic fluid and cultured amniotic fluid cells obtained from pregnancies in which the fetus has TSD.

For these reasons, TSD is the first recessive disorder which lends itself to a prospective prevention program without imposing serious restrictions on the mate selection choices of individuals or the reproductive hopes of a couple. Carrier screening among individuals of childbearing age in the defined population should permit the identification of couples at risk for TSD in their offspring. Roughly 1 in 900 couples in the Jewish population would be expected to be found at risk. Once identified and appropriately counseled, selective monitoring of all pregnancies in those identified at-risk couples could permit successful reproduction in these families and effective disease prevention at the same time.

With these considerations in mind, a voluntary, community-based, adult genetic screening program directed at the prospective prevention of this rare autosomal recessive disease was initiated in 1971 in the Baltimore-Washington areas.[11]

Voluntary screening of a healthy adult population to identify individuals who carry deleterious genes is a new concept in health care and raises complex questions. An alternative approach, mandatory (or legislated) screening, although easier to implement perhaps, was regarded as unwarranted, unnecessary and ethically unacceptable. Accordingly, it was recognized that if voluntary screening were to succeed, it would require an effective and thorough mechanism for informing and educating the public. A strategic plan was designed, therefore, to achieve this goal. The intent of this effort was clear – to inform young families accurately about a condition which most had not even heard of before, to provide clear and understandable information about how the disease could be prevented through carrier screening (blood tests) and genetic counseling, and, in so doing, to enable each couple to decide, through understanding and concern (rather than fear), whether or not to comply to the screening test.

Clearly, many important questions were recognized concerning such an effort. Could accurate and effective education of this type be delivered to a large lay community? Would such an effort create fear and unwarranted anxiety in young families? Would sufficient numbers of people respond to a public education program to make the effort meaningful with regard to effective genetic disease prevention? Inherited disease is a relatively unexplored concept for the great majority of the public. How could such information be delivered in the most meaningful and unthreatening manner?

Because of these concerns and the obvious complexity of developing an intensive communication with the community, it was recognized that the participation of important community leaders in the planning and delivery of such a program would be essential if it were to be successful. The medical, religious and organizational leadership of the Jewish communities of Baltimore and Washington, D. C., were sought out, informed and integrated into the formulation and delivery of the program. A period of 14 months, before initiating the public education testing phases of the program, was utilized for leadership education, planning and manpower organization. The details of these aspects of the program have been described elsewhere.[12]

Community Education

The education of the target community began six to eight weeks before mass screening began. Twelve community-based screening sessions were carried out in the Baltimore-Washington areas in the course of the first year of the program (in synagogues, community centers, etc.). Each of these efforts was preceded by an intensive educational program directed at a relatively specific subpopulation within the community. These included members of specific organizations, synagogue congregation members or members of the "nonaffiliated" Jewish community (reached through the press, TV, radio, etc.). Multiple educational approaches were utilized. The intent of this "saturation education effort" was to bring accurate and clear information to the community. With multiple information mechanisms, it was hoped that word-of-mouth, third-party interpretations of the "message" would be minimized. Since there were multiple means by which the information could reach a couple, it was hoped that at least one such approach would succeed. There were a number of educational mechanisms utilized: letters from rabbinical leadership to their congregants, fliers from community organizations, medical presentations in the community, telephone calls from squads of specially trained volunteers, brochures and information provided by medical practitioners and special mailings from other community leadership. The intensive educational effort was directed at either specific subpopulations or to the general public at large. For a period of four weeks prior to each testing, this educational effort was reinstituted in either the Baltimore or Washington communities.

Groups of trained volunteers from several organizations were brought together to work on each testing. From organizational membership lists as well as congregational lists, it was possible to develop a target population for each testing. In this way a carefully directed, intensive educational program could be conducted. All appropriate individuals (couples of childbearing age) in such organizations, congregations, etc. were recipients of the multifaceted educational effort.

Sociologic Considerations and the Compliance Study

Because of the unprecedented nature of this program, and because of its wide social implications, a number of selected areas for sociologic evaluation were defined. The major areas addressed by these studies were as follows:

1. The effectiveness of the educational program.
2. Factors responsible for compliance to the voluntary testing program.
3. The impact and possible stigmatization resulting from carrier identification on the individual, the couple and family, and the community-at-large.

Studies relating to the first and last of these areas are still in progress. Obviously, studies which concern the impact and stigmatization questions will require an ongoing follow-up over a prolonged period. These are being done.[13] Some data from the educational effectiveness study will be included here, but a more complete and definitive study in this area is currently being conducted.[14]

A critical study was designed to answer the important questions – who volunteers for such a test and why do they do so? And of equal significance, we wished to answer the same questions about those who do not comply. The results of this compliance study are presented in this report and have been briefly presented elsewhere.[15]

The Participants

The heterozygote screening test was available strictly on a voluntary basis. Families and individuals were informed as to the time and place of the testings. They presented themselves at the synagogue, school or community center if they wished to be tested. A two-part questionnaire was self-administered by each individual who volunteered for the test at the community facility. These forms were completed immediately before the blood sample was taken. The questionnaire was aimed at establishing a number of personal, social, family and attitudinal parameters concerning those who volunteered. In addition, certain information was obtained which would reflect the knowledge level of that person concerning the disease and the testing program. All individuals tested completed these forms. The questionnaire is illustrated in Tables 1 and 2.

The first part of the questionnaire (Table 1) provided important personal information about each person tested. In addition to his age, marital status and religious background, important questions were asked regarding his ancestry, family medical history and whether or not specific factors such as TSD or other infant death in the family might be important reasons for his desire to be tested. Also, certain medical questions were asked which might affect the accuracy of the screening test. This was also the reason for questions related to the use of various drugs and the possible effects of a recent meal. Family and pregnancy data were also collected from each person as indicated.

Part 2 of the questionnaire (Table 2) was directed at defining, in some detail, the personal and religious attitudes and health beliefs of the tested population. In addition, specific questions were asked to evaluate the effectiveness of the educational effort and which modes of education were most or least effective in reaching the public. The first four questions dealt with educational, occupational and religious attitudes of the participant. Questions 5-8 dealt with health attitudes and questions 9-14 dealt, to some extent, with the screenee's knowledge about Tay-Sachs heterozygosity and its implications for family planning. These questions related to the individual's perceived susceptibility and perceived seriousness as well.[16] That is, they asked the individual how likely he thought himself to be a

Table 1. Tay-Sachs Program Screening Questionnaire

A. No.

Date: Spouse's name:

Name: Age:

Complete address: Telephone:

Age: Religion:

Marital status: Family physician:

Wife's maiden name: Obstetrician:

B. Background

1. Country of origin of ancestors (parents or grandparents) if other than U.S.:
2. Has Tay-Sachs disease ever occurred in a blood relative?
   If so, what exact relationship?
3. Has any blood relative been identified as a Tay-Sachs carrier?
   If so, give name and exact relationship:
4. Has any blood relative died in infancy (between 1 mo. and 4 yrs.)?
   Indicate cause if known:

C. Personal History

1. Do you have any long-standing medical illness?
2. Are you diabetic? Taking Insulin?
3. Do you have any current illness?
4. Have you taken any medication in the past week? (Check twice if taken today.)
   Vitamins
   Aspirin
   Birth control pills
   (Brand: ____________________)
   Diet pills
   Other - please designate:
   Sleeping pills
   Tranquilizers
   Thyroid medication
   Antibiotics
5. How many hours since your last meal?

D. Family Facts (for woman, or man re: wife)

1. No. of pregnancies: No. of living children:
2. Any miscarriages or spontaneous abortions: Stillbirths:
3. Are you pregnant now? How many weeks?

Total hexosaminidase activity: nanamoles umbelliferone produced per hr/ml serum

Hex A:

Diagnosis: NC _____ C _____ I _____

RT NC _____ C _____

Table 2. Tay-Sachs Screening Program Confidential Questionnaire

The purpose of these questions is to evaluate the implications of this type of genetic disease prevention program. Your answers will be kept confidential and the results of this study will be presented in statistical form only, without the use of any names whatsoever. It is important that you try to answer every question as accurately as you can. In writing your answers, please do not discuss them with your spouse or anyone else. Thank you for your cooperation.

1. Circle the highest grade you completed in school:

   1 2 3 4 5 6 7 8 9 10 11 12 (High School) 13 14 15 16 (College) 17+ (Postgrad.)

2. What kind of work have you done for most of your life? (Please be specific):

   (For married men and women: What kind of work has your spouse done for most of his life?):

3. Please check your religious affiliation or preference:

   ____ Jewish Orthodox ____ Jewish Conservative ____ Jewish Reform
   Other ____________________ (Please specify)

4. To what extent do you observe religious requirements?

   ____ A great deal ____ A little
   ____ Somewhat ____ Not at all

5. Please rate your present general health (Check one):

   ____ Excellent ____ Good ____ Fair ____ Poor

6. Approximately when did you last see a doctor?

   ____ Days ago ____ Weeks ago
   ____ Months ago ____ Years ago

7. Would you say you think about your health (Check one):

   ____ Very often ____ Fairly often
   ____ Once in a while ____ Hardly ever

8. When you start to feel sick, do you usually go to a doctor right away, or do you usually wait a day or so to see what happens?

   ____ Usually go right away ____ Usually wait and see

9. How likely do you think it is that <u>you</u> might be a Tay-Sachs carrier?

   ____ Hardly likely ____ Somewhat likely
   ____ Fairly likely ____ Very likely

10. What is the likelihood that a Jewish person of central-eastern European background is a carrier of the gene for Tay-Sachs disease?

    ____ 1 in 3,600 ____ 1 in 900
    ____ 1 in 30 ____ 1 in 10

11. If you or your spouse (only one) were found to be a Tay-Sachs carrier, how much do you feel it would matter to you?

    ____ A great deal ____ A moderate amount
    ____ Somewhat ____ Hardly at all

12. Do you plan to have any (additional) children?

    ____ Yes ____ No

    (If no, please go to question 13.)

Table 2. (Continued)

A. Suppose you or your spouse were found to be a Tay-Sachs carrier. How do you feel that would affect your plans for having (additional) children? (Check one)

____ I would not change my plans for having (additional) children.
____ I would still have (additional) children, but fewer than I planned before.
____ I would decide not to have any (additional) children.
____ Other (please specify): ____________

B. Suppose you and your spouse were found to be Tay-Sachs carriers, how would that affect your plans for having (addidional) children?

____ I would not change my plans for having (additional) children.
____ I would still have (additional children, but fewer than I planned before.
____ I would decide not to have any (additional) children.
____ Other (please specify): ____________

13. Suppose you (your wife) were pregnant, and medical tests around the fourth month showed that the fetus had Tay-Sachs disease. On balance, would you guess that you would favor or not favor medically terminating the pregnancy?

____ Would favor ____ Would not favor

14. While a decision involving abortion involves many aspects of life, would you say that, FOR YOU, the major basis for the decision would be on: (Check one)

____ Medical grounds ____ Religious doctrine ____ Personal philosophy

15. About how long ago did you first learn of the Tay-Sachs screening program?

____ Past week ____ Past month
____ Past few months ____ More than a few months ago

16. How did you first learn of the Tay-Sachs screening program? (Check one)

____ TV or radio ____ Newspaper ____ Relative ____ Friend
____ Temple (meetings, newsletter, etc.) ____ Acquaintance ____ Other

17. Did you try to obtain further information about the program?

____ Yes ____ No If yes, from whom: ____ Friend ____ Relative
____ Doctor ____ Rabbi ____ Other ____ Tay-Sachs Program

18. Did you tell others about the program?

____ Yes ____ No If yes, whom (Please give names):
____ Relatives (specify relationships and names):
____ Friends ____ Acquaintances (list names and relationships on the back of this paper)

19. Did anyone suggest that you not participate in this program?

____ Yes ____ No ____ If yes, who: ____ Friend ____ Doctor
____ Rabbi ____ Relative

20. What was the major reason that led you to participate in this program?

____
____

21. Did you at any time have any misgivings about participating in this program?

____ Yes ____ No ____ If yes, what were they? ____________
____

I consent to have a blood sample taken from me to determine if I carry the gene for Tay-Sachs disease. I understand that all of the information which I have provided, as well as the results of my test, will be handled confidentially and that the information may be used for statistical purposes only.

Signature: ____________

carrier of the TSD gene and how serious it would be if he were. The remaining questions related to the diffusion of information in the community and to the ways people received information.[17] The possibility of negative attitudes in the community was also addressed.

After the completion of the first eight testings (including three in greater Washington and five in the Baltimore area), a random selection of 500 participant questionnaire sets was made. This provided the sample from which the compliant data are derived. All questionnaires were anonymously coded, key-punched and the data placed on programmed computer tapes.

The Nonparticipants

As previously indicated, the nature of the educational program was to saturate a selected population of childbearing-age couples with specific information immediately before a community testing session. It could be readily ascertained from available lists, therefore, which individuals had received the educational program but had not presented for testing. This mechanism provided access to a substantial number of noncompliants. From these, a random selection was made of 500 nonparticipants. A mailing was made to these individuals which included an explanatory covering letter, the identical two-part questionnaire which the participants had completed and a stamped return envelope. The recipients were asked to complete the questionnaires and to return them to the program. Within a two- to three-month period after the mailing, 412 nonparticipants (82% of the sample) complied with this request. Their forms were processed in identical fashion to that used for the participant sample.

Results

In the first year of the program, 12 community-based testings were conducted. In that period 6,938 individuals volunteered for the TSD carrier-detection test. (An additional 3,000 persons have since been tested in the Baltimore-Washington areas.) The detailed results of these efforts have been reported elsewhere.[12] In the first year, over 300 individuals were found to carry the gene for TSD (approximately 1 in 24 tested). Importantly, 11 at-risk couples were identified in this sample, none of whom had previously had a TSD child. Five pregnancies have occurred in this group since identification; all couples chose to monitor their pregnancies, and one was electively aborted after a positive intrauterine diagnosis was made. The diagnosis was definitively corroborated in the aborted fetus.[18]

Demographic Factors

The composition of the tested population is tabulated in Table 3. In the first year 56% of those tested were female and 44% male. This difference was even more marked than is apparent, since approximately 280 men were tested whose wives could not be, due to pregnancy at the time of the testing. (Pregnancy interferes with the screening test.) Of those tested 94% were married, 5% were engaged and only 1% were single. This clearly reflects a "program bias." Single individuals were counseled in detail as to the "program preference" of testing married or engaged couples. Approximately 90% of the single people who came for testing and who were counseled, decided to wait until after marriage to have the test performed. Approximately 70% of the married individuals were tested as couples.

The sex and age distribution of the tested individuals are shown in Table 4. It is of considerable interest that a marked skew toward the younger age group is apparent in both the male and female groups. An even younger age distribution among females, compared with males, probably reflects the younger age of females at the time of marriage. The striking predominance of young married couples noted in the voluntarily tested population is very significant and highly relevant to the compliance studies conducted. Further comment will be made in the discussion section of this paper.

The educational level among the participants was extraordinarily high (as might be expected in this ethnic group). With data evaluated from two random testings (1,102 persons), it can be seen in Table 5 that nearly 75% of those tested had completed college and 43% had some postgraduate education. The implications of this will also be discussed later.

Although the carrier detection test was available to all individuals, the thrust of the public education program was in the Jewish community. It would appear, from Table 6, that the appropriate community was represented in those coming for the test. Again, the data are derived from two representative testings of the 12 which were conducted. Certain differences in the compositions of the Jewish communities of Baltimore vs. Washington are not reflected in this Table since the data have been combined. These differences, however, are not relevant for the purposes here. Of those tested 94% indicated they were Jewish. The proportions of Reformed, Conservative and Orthodox were approximately representative (Associated Jewish Charities of Baltimore and Washington, personal communication). Different religious backgrounds were indicated by 3.4% (almost all were married to Jewish individuals), and 3% did not specify what religious group they belonged to or did not answer.

Table 3. Demographic Factors of Individuals Screened in Voluntary Tay-Sachs Disease Carrier Detection Program*

	%	*No.*
Females	56	3,886
Males	44**	3,052
Married	94	
Engaged	5	
Single	1	

*Based on first 12 screening sessions (6,938 persons).

**Two hundred eighty males were tested whose wives were untested because of current pregnancy.

Table 4. Sex and Age Distribution of Individuals Screened in Voluntary TSD Carrier Testing Program*

	Males		*Females*	
	No.	*%*	*No.*	*%*
20 yrs.	6	0.2	524	13.5
20-24 yrs.	740	24.2	1,328	34.2
25-29 yrs.	1,062	34.8	1,367	35.2
30-34 yrs.	720	23.6	388	9.9
35-39 yrs.	280	9.2	159	4.1
40+ yrs.	244	8.0	120	3.1
Total	3,052	100.0	3,886	100.0

*Based on first 12 testings (6,938 persons).

Table 5. Educational Level Among Participants in Voluntary Tay-Sachs Screening Program*

Highest Completed Year of Education	*No.*	*% of Total*
1 through 8	2	0.2
9 through 11	5	0.5
Grade 12	85	7.7
13 through 15	194	17.6
College grad.	334	30.3
Postgrad study	473	42.9
No answer	9	0.8
Total	1,102	100.0

*Data accumulated from two testings (one in Baltimore, one in Washington area).

Compliance Analyses

A comparison was made of the data derived from questionnaires completed by 500 randomly selected individuals who voluntarily came for testing with those from 412 (of 500) nonparticipants who returned the same questionnaires which had been mailed to them. A coded number system (1 = lowest, 4 = highest) was used for scoring answers to those questions where a numerical answer itself was not given by the respondent. All statistical analyses were made using Student's t-test and differences were considered to be significant if $p < 0.05$. In Tables 7 and 8 variables between the participant and nonparticipant groups are compared. Table 7 lists the data concerning those variables where definite, statistically significant, differences were found. No significant differences between the two groups were found where the variables listed in Table 8 were compared.

The participants were significantly younger, had fewer children, were less likely to have completed their families (74% of the compliants indicated plans for further children compared with 21% of the non-compliants), and were better educated than the nonparticipant group. Using the Hollingshead scale for social position,[17] the participants ranked higher.

Turning to an analysis of those questions which dealt primarily with the knowledge level of the individuals and their perception and attitude toward the information provided, several striking and important differences were noted. When asked to indicate the likelihood of being a carrier, the participants indicated a higher susceptibility than the nonparticipant groups. On the other hand, when asked questions about the seriousness of being a carrier, the noncompliants indicated a significantly greater concern as to the seriousness of such a discovery.

When asked how the finding that one member of the couple was a carrier would affect future plans for children, those who complied and were tested were much less likely to alter their plans. If both parents were found to be carriers, the compliants again were significantly less likely to change their reproductive plans than the nonparticipating group. However, the participants *did* indicate a change by reducing the number of children they would have or by stating that they would use "other" approaches if both were found to be carriers. In nearly all instances where the participants indicated "other," they explained that they would elect to use the fetal diagnostic test in order to still have children.

The questions relating to change in family planning as a function of heterozygote detection in one or both members of the couple clearly indicate a greater understanding of the genetic implications of hetero-

Table 6. Religious Affiliation Among Participants in Baltimore-Washington Tay-Sachs Screening Program*

Affiliation	*No.*	*% of Total*
Jewish Reformed	323	29.3
Jewish Conservative	576	52.3
Jewish Orthodox	132	12.0
Other (religion specified)	38	3.4
Other (no religion specified)	16	1.5
No answer	17	1.5
Total	1,102	100.0

*Data accumulated from two testings (one in Baltimore, one in Washington area).

Table 7. Tay-Sachs Screening Program: Compliance Factors

Variable	*Participants* *Mean Score*	*No.*	*Nonparticipants* *Mean Score*	*No.*	*t-Test* *Sign at 0.05*
Age	27.70	491	34.90	407	Yes
No. pregnancies	0.96	423	2.30	386	Yes
No. living children	0.77	417	1.97	385	Yes
Yrs. education completed*	7.24	489	6.97	410	Yes
Index of social position	72.10	452	70.90	407	Yes
**Perceived susceptibility	1.65	460	1.38	379	Yes
**Perceived seriousness	2.94	485	3.19	405	Yes
Change family plans, if					
**Either carrier	1.25	356	1.72	95	Yes
**Both carriers	1.81	325	2.41	85	Yes

*Beyond the 8th grade.
**Coded scale: 1 = lowest, 4 = highest.

Table 8. Tay-Sachs Screening Program: Compliance Study

Variable	*Participants* *Mean Score**	*No.*	*Nonparticipants* *Mean Score**	*No.*	*t-Test* *Sign at 0.05*
Degree of religiosity	2.45	486	2.48	411	No
Perceived health status	1.41	492	1.47	411	No
Last visit to MD	2.16	491	2.16	411	No
Frequency think about health	2.44	489	2.50	409	No
No. of meds.	1.11	492	1.07	412	No

*Coded Scale: 1 = lowest, 4 = highest.

zygosity among those complying to the Tay-Sachs test. It was significantly better understood by the participants that if *one* member of the couple were proved a carrier, there would be little concern for disease in their offspring. This is reflected by the relatively minimal indication to change family plans in that situation among the participant group. The nonparticipants, on the other hand, perceived the seriousness of heterozygosity in one member of the couple quantitatively greater than the participant group. This may be interpreted as a lack of thorough understanding of the educational material provided. Where the supposition was presented that both members of the couple would be found to be carriers, again it could be interpreted that the nonparticipants showed less thorough understanding of the educational material, in that a much higher percentage indicated they would not have further children nor would they use other means (such as amniocentesis) in order to complete their planned family.

A number of important comparisons showed no significant differences between the participant and nonparticipant groups. These are catalogued in Table 8. No significant differences existed between the two groups with regard to their religious attitudes, their personal health standards nor the frequency with which they thought about their health or used medications. Similar comparisons of the responses to questions concerning attitudes toward abortion indicated no significant differences between the compliants and noncompliants on this issue.

Discussion and Conclusions

The major differences, therefore, between the participant and nonparticipant groups were their age, their current family size and, importantly, their plans for further children. The last difference is highly significant ($p \ll 0.05$) and may be *the* critical factor which permits formation of a hypothesis to explain the other observed differences.

If individuals are to adopt health-benefiting innovations, it may *require* that some clear and specific incentive be established by which individuals will be prompted to adopt such behavior. A genetic testing program like that described has primary implications for the reproductive future of a couple. Therefore, the incentive to carefully evaluate and appreciate educational material and testing of this type would most likely exist in this group. The marked skew toward the younger age distribution in the tested population most probably reflects the desire for future children in this group. The predominance of women volunteering for the test may also reflect a greater concern in them about matters concerning future children than in men (or that they are less fearful of blood tests).

The small percentage of families in later reproductive years who volunteered for testing may well indicate that there was not sufficient incentive in this age group (where most had completed their families) to volunteer for a blood test of this type. If the couple has completed its reproduction, there might be little reason to carefully evaluate (and thereby to understand), the educational information provided by the program. This creates a situation where lesser understanding (and perhaps greater misconceptions) is likely to result.

One of the more remarkable findings in these data is the intriguing difference between the perceived susceptibility and the perceived seriousness of being a carrier between the two groups. In many public health programs it is regarded that the susceptibility of the individual must be perceived as high in order to elicit a positive health response from the individual. In addition, the perception of seriousness must also be enhanced for an appropriate response. In our study the participants showed a higher perceived susceptibility but a lesser perceived seriousness than the nonparticipants. One might speculate that the latter, not understanding as well, misconceived certain vital information (increased seriousness of being a carrier) and then used denial to avoid inner conflicts (decreased susceptibility).

Without an incentive for critical evaluation and understanding of the health information provided, the couple in which further family reproduction is unlikely may less well appreciate the new health information provided. Since the program was heavily oriented to the concept that families could still reproduce, even if found to be at risk, it is reasonable that in the community this was a program which identified mainly with families planning further children. The younger age group heavily represented in the tested population supports this concept.

If people understand less well, they are likely to have greater misconceptions. In a reproductive sense, if only one member of the couple is a carrier of this recessive gene, there should be no hazard with regard to reproduction. Here the nonparticipants may have misconceived this information since they indicated that they would change, reduce or cease further reproduction if one member of the couple were found to be a carrier far more commonly than the participant group. If both members were carriers, again the nonparticipants showed a much greater likelihood to stop reproduction completely, and not nearly so often indicated the use of amniocentesis as a means for still being able to reproduce.

Several interesting comparisons in this study showed *no* differences between participants and nonparticipants. While it was a concern of the program at its inception that Orthodox Jews might be less inclined to participate in genetic screening of this kind because of their more conservative position on abortion, the distribution among compliants and noncompliants was nearly identical with regard to religious affiliation. In both groups approximately 15%-20% indicated Orthodox Jewish background. With regard to attitudes toward abortion and toward aborting fetuses with TSD, again no differences were found. More than 90% indicated that they would terminate pregnancy where a Tay-Sachs fetus was identified.

The heavy emphasis in the educational program on providing reproductive information with positive reproductive alternatives, regardless of genotype designation, would appear to have been moderately successful. Since the overwhelming distribution of people who came for the testing was young couples planning further reproduction, it is implied that this message did, in fact, reach them. The responses to questions dealing with reproduction indicate that nearly 100% of those tested would elect to use amniocentesis as a reproductive alternative if they were found to be at risk. Moreover, the termination of a pregnancy in which the fetus was found to have Tay-Sachs disease was uniformly regarded as a reasonable alternative.

The great majority of those who volunteered for testing indicated plans for future children. This fact should be considered if a true compliance figure to the test is to be determined. Although nearly 60,000 people between 18 and 45 years of age were estimated in the Jewish communities of Baltimore and Washington, it is possible that only a third (or 20,000) would be couples planning further children. If this assumption is correct, the compliance in the first one to two years of the voluntary heterozygote screening program in these areas may be as high as 50%. It is concluded that an effective and intense educational program directed at the prevention of an untreatable genetic disease, which simultaneously provides positive reproductive alternatives for all couples, can elicit a significant response from a highly educated, health-oriented, organized and cooperative community. Its overall value will have to await the completion of other psychosocial studies. For many reasons, this approach to the prevention of Tay-Sachs disease, in this community, may provide the optimal model for evaluating such mechanisms for the prospective prevention of inherited diseases. Much of what we learn in principle and design may have important implications for other voluntary genetic disease prevention programs in other communities in the future.

Acknowledgments

The efforts of Drs. Barton Childs, Norman Scotch, Sol Levine, David McQueen, Neil Holtzman and Haig Kazazian, Jr. are gratefully acknowledged.

References

1. Carter, C. O., Fraser-Roberts, J. A., Evans, K. A. et al: Genetic clinic: A follow-up. *Lancet, 1*:281, 1971.
2. Myrianthopoulos, N. C. and Aronson, S. M.: Population dynamics of Tay-Sachs disease. *Amer. J. Hum. Genet., 18*:313, 1966.
3. Leonard, C. O., Chase, G. A. and Childs, B.: Genetic counseling: A consumer's view. *New Eng. J. Med., 287*:433, 1972.
4. Hsia, D. Y.: The detection of heterozygous carriers. *Med. Clin. N. Amer., 53*:857, 1969.
5. Brady, R. O., Johnson, W. G. and Uhlendorf, B. W.: Identification of heterozygous carriers of lipid storage diseases. *Amer. J. Med., 51*:423, 1971.
6. Kaback, M. M. and Zeiger, R. S.: Heterozygote detection in Tay-Sachs disease: A prototype community screening program for the prevention of recessive genetic disorders. In Volk and Aronson (eds.): *Advances in Experimental Medicine and Biology*. New York:Plenum Press, 1972, vol. 19, p. 613.
7. Aronson, S. M.: Epidemiology. In Volk, B. W. (ed.): *Tay-Sachs Disease,* New York:Grune and Stratton, Inc., 1964.
8. O'Brien, J. S., Okada, S., Chen, A. and Fillerup, D. L.: Tay-Sachs disease. Detection of heterozygotes and homozygotes by serum hexosaminidase assay. *New Eng. J. Med., 283*:15, 1970.
9. Schneck, L., Valenti, C., Amsterdam, D. et al: Prenatal diagnosis of Tay-Sachs disease. *Lancet, 1*:582, 1970.
10. O'Brien, J. S., Okada, S., Fillerup, D. L. et al: Tay-Sachs disease: Prenatal diagnosis. *Science, 172*:61, 1971.
11. Kaback, M. M. and O'Brien, J. S.: Tay-Sachs: Prototype for prevention of genetic disease. *Hosp. Prac. 8*:107-116, 1973.
12. Kaback, M. M., Zeiger, R. S., Reynolds, L. W. and Sonneborn, M.: Approaches to the prevention and control of Tay-Sachs disease. In Steinberg, A. G. and Bearn, A. G. (eds.): *Progress in Medical Genetics.* New York:Academic Press, vol. 10. (In press.)
13. Gordis, L., Childs, B. and Kaback, M.: (In preparation.)
14. Kaback, M. M. and Greenwald, S.: (In preparation.)
15. Kaback, M. M., Ruth, M. V. and Becker, M. H.: Compliance factors in a voluntary heterozygote screening program. Abstract, *Amer. J. Hum. Gen.,* 1973. (In press.)
16. Rosenstock, I. M.: Why people use health services. *Milbank Mem. Fund. Quart., 44* (no. 3, part 2):94, 1966.
17. McQueen, D. V.: *Genetic Screening,* thesis. The Johns Hopkins University School of Public Health, Baltimore, 1972.
18. Kaback, M. M., Thomas, G. and Holtzman, N. A.: (In preparation.)

Some Social and Psychologic Issues in Genetic Screening

Public and Professional Adaptation to Biomedical Innovation

James R. Sorenson, Ph.D.

Introduction

The title of this article is meant to suggest three points which are worth noting at the beginning. First, this discussion will address itself to some social and psychologic issues which may arise with the advent of genetic screening. These issues include such things as possible stigmatization which may accompany carrier status identification and the possible social, economic and political discrimination which may ensue. Such potential developments could be labeled as risks, risks that individuals and the public may face in acceptance of screening as routine medical practice or as the product of legislative enactments. However, the word risk connotes perhaps too much of a value bias and in so doing exposes the strongly held values involved in the application of the science of genetics to the problems of men. Some may consider reduction in marriage chances that a person may face as a result of being identified as a carrier of a defective gene as a good thing, since it could reduce the occurrence of specific diseases in the population. Others would consider this such a serious compromise of the individual's right to a complete and full social life that the risk of reduced marriageability outweighs the benefits which could result from carrier status identification. Still others would want to note this as a possible issue arising from genetic screening and to consider how the benefits offered by screening may be realized and any unintended consequences worked through. In the discussion which follows, we will

---

James R. Sorenson, Ph.D., *Assistant Professor, Department of Sociology, Princeton University, Princeton, N. J.*

attempt to navigate a course of inquiry and hypothesis formulation that follows the third path. In suggesting possible social and psychologic issues which may arise, we do so not in the spirit of viewing with alarm, but rather with the intent of providing a more rounded view of genetic screening as a sociopsychologic event.

Second, the title is intended to suggest that adaptation rather than adoption is the most fruitful way of viewing the advent of genetic screening. While adoption connotes the idea of ready acceptance and to some degree a lack of problems in implementation, adaptation suggests that problems exist in application, problems which can be solved by a give-and-take exchange between the experts and the public. Thus, in opposition to viewing the utilization of screening from the perspective of a passive receptive audience and an active, forceful body of experts, we are going to view issues in genetic screening from a more dynamic perspective, where all concerned must expect to adjust their views and expectations. As is the case with almost any biomedical development, the benefits which accrue from applying genetic screening to man are not absolute or without cost. While there may be strong sentiment to apply such a development as rapidly as possible because of health benefits, the application imperative inherent in scientific and technologic developments should be weighed in light of the costs which may accompany such use. It would seem that our use of developments with the potential impact of applied human genetics should be premised on a more critically evaluative approach. While we have devoted vast sums of money and intellectual resources to developing a battery of biomedical devices which can help man biologically, we have given little attention to devising ways of evaluating our use of such developments. Examination of such issues may serve as a beginning in developing social arrangements which insure more effective use of biomedical innovations.

Third, the title is meant to suggest that the social and psychologic issues in the use of genetic screening are matters of concern to both the public and the professionals involved. Our society is certainly moving in the direction of becoming more and more a knowledgeable society. By this we mean that to an increasing degree individuals and society are finding themselves dependent on various experts for information and assistance in arriving at solutions to problems. While the expertise of the professional may qualify him to provide comment on the scientific aspects of a problem, this expertise does not necessarily qualify him to make pronouncements on whether the problem, in fact, ought to be solved or just how society might go about solving it. Our current social mechanisms for filtering knowledge from science into society via the professional, and in the process granting the professional considerable discretion in how to use this knowledge, may be a social invention which is in need of considerable revision. Of course, the public's orientation to knowledge utilization, whether in medicine or any other area, must correspondingly undergo change – change which makes the public a more willing and active partner in developing adaptations to biomedical developments. While an examination of this topic is certainly beyond the scope of the current paper, the issues are all present in genetic screening.

Finally, of the various types of issues that may be associated with genetic screening, we have selected only a small set for examination. Attention is given in this paper to some of the social and psychologic issues which screening may pose for the individual, for husband and wife and for the extended family in this society. In contrast to the wealth of literature on the scientific and ethical issues involved in genetic screening, we will address man less as a scientific or ethical decision maker and more as a sociopsychologic actor. By this we mean that our attention will be given primarily to examining how genetic screening may affect individual feelings of personal worth as well as its possible impact on the establishment of, or the maintenance of, established social relationships. A basic premise of the discussion to follow will be that we can best appreciate the social psychology of genetic screening by keeping in mind the idea that what is involved in learning that one is the carrier of a deleterious gene is not just the acquisition of this knowledge. Rather, the meaning of being identified as a carrier resides in the ways in which the information maintains or alters how the individual views himself both as an integral person and as a social creature. It is through the establishment of such a meaning that the significance of genetic screening and carrier status identification will eventually exhibit itself in health and reproductive behavior.

A Brief Historical Sketch

Man has been aware of gross observable inborn differences between individuals for ages. Awareness of differences has only recently expanded to include not only highly accurate prediction of when such events occur but also measurement and prediction of subtle, nonobservable, genetic differences. These developments have expanded tremendously the practical significance of human genetics. A brief examination of the historical setting of applied human genetics in this society will prove useful by the light it sheds on current cultural attitudes and values toward genetic abnormalities.

In this society, widespread practical interest in human genetics has been limited largely to two historical periods. The first interest in applied genetics occurred in the age of reform, during the late 1800s and early 1900s.[1] Applied genetics in this era was lodged within the more general cultural movement of social reform and human betterment.[2] In this context, applied genetics found itself in the domain of experts in social reform, and human genetics was seen as a solution to an array of social problems. The most recent interest in human genetics witnesses a significant transition from this earlier period. Today genetics is no longer lodged within a cultural movement of social reform and human betterment, but rather is rapidly becoming a subfield within medicine,* the domain of experts in clinical practice.[3,4]

In a broad historical sense, this basic shift signals several important changes in the purpose, scope and impact of genetics in American society and also conditions the meanings attached to our increasing capacity to measure genetic variability. During the earlier period applied genetics, couched in the language of social problems, saw such issues as biologic and social eugenics, racial fitness and the ideal-type man become central, if perhaps unexamined, concepts directing the social significance of genetic variability. This was the era of eugenics, and with the eugenicists' prediction of an eventual genetic apocalypse, applied genetics seemed a necessity if the dire forecasts of the eugenicists were to be avoided. People suffering from genetic misfortune, both those phenotypically afflicted as well as those suspected to be carriers of undesirable traits, were viewed as problems. Many saw such people as the basic cause of existing social ills, as threats to the maintenance of society. And, many saw in them the seeds of the eugenicists' concern.[5]

Applied genetics within the confines of clinical medicine today exhibits some very significant divergences from these earlier concerns.

---

*Applied genetics within medicine is limited today largely to what can be called physician-investigators rather than general family doctors. As with most biomedical inventions, diffusion of developments within the medical sphere begins with the medical personnel who bridge the gap between scientific research and clinical practice. Their involvement in the world of science as well as the domain of medicine makes them particularly well qualified to act as trendsetters in shaping routine medicine's use of science. In discussing the developing role of human genetics in medicine it must be stressed that most of the comments we will be making are in reference to physician-investigators rather than the more common family doctor. The newness of human genetics as a clinical issue and the sparse genetic training most physicians receive in medical school limit clinical genetics largely to physician-investigators. A recent survey of general physicians in Massachusetts by Albrecht and Day[3] confirms this observation by noting that over two thirds of the family doctors surveyed seldom or never provided genetic services or counseling to their patients.

Within the context of medicine genetic problems, both phenotypic disease as well as carrier status, are seen less, if at all, as social threats and more as individual or family problems. The concern of the doctor in clinical genetics is most often the individual family and their disease, not society. The basic orientation of most doctors appears to be on the reduction of disease occurrence, not improvement of the human gene pool. Doctors, in their application of modern human genetics, most often put the interests and desires of the family ahead of concerns about the possible social significance of genetically defective people marrying and reproducing.[6]* Whereas the patient during the eugenic era was society, and the problem was preventing social ills, today the patient is most often an individual or a married couple, and the problem is disease avoidance.

The movement of applied genetics from the province of social problem to that of medicine, and more specifically from concern with racial purity to disease elimination, is not complete. Some still express considerable concern about the human gene pool and view the human genetic condition from the perspective of preservation of current levels of genetic health or improvement of the human gene pool through various eugenic measures.[7,8] Nevertheless, the most immediate and practical aspects of applied genetics today are occurring largely within the confines of the medical world, and most uses, actual and potential, are couched in terms of disease control and elimination.

Genetics in Medicine: Genetic Health and Genetic Disease

In American society human genetics is applied in only a few ways, but it has promise of much wider application.[9] Within the medical world, in

*This is not to say that there is no concern within the medical profession for the long-term impact of medical treatment. There is, as witnessed by the recent Stevenson and Howell article.[6] The argument presented here simply suggests that with the movement of applied genetics from the realm of social problem to clinical medicine, the social arrangements of professional medicine, and in particular the doctor-patient relationship, make it incumbent on the doctor, at least ideally, to put the interests and concerns of his patients above those of society. This is in sharp contrast to the social reformers who were at the forefront of applied genetics during the eugenics era. No such social arrangement was operating then, and the view social reformers took on applying what was then known about genetics was from the perspective of society. Accordingly, the individual and his rights were at times seriously compromised so the interests of society, as defined by the social reformers, could be maintained. It is perhaps instructive to note that one could claim that many see the new genetics as a social problem. However, it must be pointed out that what is taken now as problematic is not a set of social issues that the new genetics may be able to solve, but rather issues revolving about the social control of the new genetics itself.

addition to the treatment of phenotypic disease, genetic knowledge is used in genetic counseling and genetic screening. While the redefinition of applied human genetics as a legitimate concern of the medical profession is not yet complete, the transition has centered the focus of applied genetics in the world of disease, and there are developing professional as well as public conceptions of genetic disease and abnormality. The eventual use of genetics in medicine and by society will be highly conditioned by the public and professional meanings which become attached to genetic variation. Of particular concern for understanding the developing role of applied genetics and genetic screening in American society, then, is an appreciation of health in this culture, and the evolving meaning of genetic variation with regard to health.

As several commentators have noted, our society exhibits sustained concern with health.[10] Health is seen as a precondition for an even more important and highly held value, individual achievement. One's achievement is threatened unless one is healthy. As has also been noted, illness can sometimes be used as a device which legitimates the lack of personal achievement. Regardless of the exact relationship between health and achievement, health, somatic and supposedly genetic as well, maintains high priority.

The conceptions of health, public as well as professional, are varied and complex. Of basic significance to these varied formulations, however, is the premise that health is essentially individual functional adequacy.[11] Health, in a general sense, is a condition in which a person can fulfill the normal routine expectations placed on him. By and large, health is defined not by holding up the strictest requirements and demanding perfection in meeting routine expectations, but rather by noting satisfactory performance. Of course, there is tremendous variation in what constitutes satisfactory functional performance but the emphasis is on minimal, not maximal performance.

Health as functional adequacy can be divided into three, more specific components which reveal the complexity of the concept. Health can be thought of in terms of physical, psychologic and social adequacy.[11] It is possible for these components to vary independently of each other, as when a person has a physical disorder, such as a minor cold, which does not affect either his psychologic or social functioning. Such variation suggests the utility of making a distinction between illness and disability.[12] Illness, which may involve altered physical, psychologic or social capacities, may not affect or result in disabilities. In fact, one of the most important duties of the health professional is defining the interrelationships among physical, psychologic and social illness and assisting the individual and society in controlling the extent to which any one illness may result in a disability. Disabilities, of course, may be directly induced by an illness, as when polio cripples an athlete, or they may be the result of social convention, as when attitudes and beliefs about blindness result in definitions of the blind as more disabled than in fact they are.[13] In the discussion which follows, it will be useful to keep the various distinctions introduced here in mind, for they can shed light on the evolving meanings of the genetic variability exposed by genetic screening as illness and the developing conceptions of carrier status as disabling.

Illness can be conceptualized as one form of social deviance and, as such, is subject to a set of social constraints. From a sociologic position, perhaps the most significant fact about illness is that it normally exempts individuals from many of the ordinary routines of social life. That is, depending on the nature of the illness, an individual may be excused and at times is kept from performing many social roles, including work, the demands of interpersonal obligations and the normal expectations of family living. Being ill, however, does not remove one from all obligations. Illness sets into motion another set of expectations, which if not performed reasonably well, incur social sanctions. For example, in the American culture the sick role normally necessitates removal from some, if not all, routine role obligations, requires realization that the sick individual cannot be expected to take care of himself, specifies that the individual must desire to get well, and demands that the sick individual seek legitimate medical advice and cooperate with medical experts in returning himself to a healthy state.[10] The lack of fulfillment of any of these behaviors can incur social censure – as when a sick person works as usual, or when he personally ministers to his illness, or expresses a desire not to get well or, perhaps most seriously, does not seek legitimate medical assistance. Of course, the demands which the sick role incur are conditioned in part by the subcultural meanings of illness as well as by the nature of the illness. If illness is of a short duration and an acute intensity, perhaps most of the above obligations apply. However, in the case of chronic or terminal illness, some of the above obligations may not.[14]

Not only are there general sets of expectations for sick individuals, but there are specific connotations associated with various diseases which refine the social meaning of illness. These connotations are often negative and result in the rejection of such people by the healthy. For example, in this culture a considerable body of research suggests that many common diseases can be ranked in terms of their relative degrees of social acceptability. In general, physical, noncosmetic disabilities (such as asthma and ulcers) are more acceptable than sensory disabilities (such as deafness and blindness), which tend to be more acceptable than cosmetic physical disabilities (such as amputation and old age), which in turn are generally more acceptable than brain injury or psychogenetic disorders (such as mental retardation and alcoholism).[15]

Disorders not only vary consistently in terms of their social acceptability, but research suggests that the amount of prejudice expressed toward physically and mentally disabled people is generally more severe than that expressed toward various minority groups.[16] Thus, to be ill, even to be legitimately ill as when one has a disease diagnosed by qualified medical personnel, is to incur various types of social stigmatization and to be perceived as more or less disabled. This stigma can lead to various forms of discrimination, some personal, some social, some political and some economic. Perhaps the most pervasive discrimination is that growing out of cultural attitudes and stereotypes of various ill and disabled people which routinizes encounters between the disabled and "normals." It is in such situations that the disabled often find it necessary to enact the culturally expected set of behaviors which normals impute to them, and in the process reinforce cultural stereotypes and perhaps significantly shape personal notions of worth, value and wholeness as a human being.

In regard to genetic diseases, it appears that they too can be ranked in terms of their social acceptability. That is, genetic disorders which impair physical function in a noncosmetic way are perhaps the most acceptable in this culture, such as diabetes, followed by genetic disorders which alter sensory functioning, followed by genetic or chromosomal anomalies which effect cosmetic physical disorders and, finally, the least acceptable are genetic or chromosomal disorders which impair mental functioning, such as mental retardation. Research on both genetic and nongenetic disorders suggests that the dimensions of a disorder which appear to most potently affect cultural responses, and in the process provide for stigmatization, are (1) visibility, that is, a disorder's degree of overtness; (2) the physicalness, its degree of physical as opposed to mental handicap; (3) social disruption, that is, the degree to which the disorder disrupts the normal routine of social life; and (4) fear, or the degree to which there may be harm to the nondisabled as a function of the disabling problem.[16]

To the extent that a given disease scores high on these dimensions, there is a significant chance that the disorder can have such serious and pervasive social impact for the affected that the individual may organize a significant portion, if not his total life around the disorder. An illness can thus serve as an organizing motif in a person's life, eclipsing the more usual organizing activities of family and work. To the degree that a disease scores low, there is a reduced chance that it will come to serve as a central organizing vehicle for the individual and hence be less disabling for the person. Instead, it may become a problem which the person learns to handle with varying degrees of success.

Identification of Carriers of Genetic Disease

Having looked at health formulations in the American culture, and in particular at the social meaning of illness, we will now examine carrier status as a health issue and its evolving meaning in both the medical and public mind.

Within the general area of medical screening our attention will be given to screening for carriers of genetic disease, not screening for the actual disease status itself. The primary function of genetic screening is to identify those individuals who have identifiable genetic carrier status and to inform such individuals or their guardians of the appropriate risk for the occurrence of genetic disease in their children. As suggested above, the meaning of being a carrier of a genetic disease is in the process of being formulated in this culture. From a broad historical perspective the meaning of hereditary problems has shifted from animistic interpretations, with their attendant locus of responsibility in the moral activity of the individual, to more naturalistic interpretations. Within this latter framework personal efficacy as a causative agent in the event has been lessened. Accordingly, there has been a reduction in the sense of both individual and societal burden attached to the occurrence of hereditary problems in a family, at least at a very general level.

With the increasing identification of applied genetics as the proper subject of the medical profession and its developing definition as a health issue, we are interested in conceptions of the carrier state as a disease or illness status and in the resulting disabilities – physical, psychologic and social – which may or may not ensue from such a status.

The physical health significance of carrier status in terms of body functioning is apparently very small. While there is some medical uncertainty over the physical health significance of some carrier states, general medical opinion suggests that there are no physical consequences which entail curtailing routine activities for carriers.[17] To be a carrier of a genetic disorder does not mean bodily illness or disability in the more routine sense of these words. With few exceptions, carrier status does not carry with it any observable public indices of being different as does the actual disease state. Recognition of carrier status has been and continues to be more often under the control of the carrier than is phenotypic disease status in general. Thus its significance for social life is more dependent on the meaning and significance of the status for the carrier individual than is the situation with disorders having public exposure. Carrier status generally constitutes a hidden dimension to overall general individual health which, until recently, has been irrelevant to most routine social intercourse. Accordingly, the significance of carrier status resides more in what it means for the individual in terms of his psychologic and social functioning.

In pursuing the psychologic and social issues which carrier status identification may entail, we will examine its significance for personal conceptions of worth and integrity and how these conceptions may affect the establishment of routine social relationships. In addition, our discussion will include examination of some possible issues which may arise when carrier status disclosure takes place in families and its significance for established social relationships. In general, a major thesis of the following discussion will be that although the state of being a carrier of a genetic disease does not constitute any personal illness risk to the carrier in the classic meaning of the word, identification as a carrier in fact may entail considerable potential for disabilities to develop – disabilities resulting not from the actual physical carrier status condition, but from the personal and social meanings which may become attached to carrier status.

Genetic Screening, Personal Identity and Social Relationships

A basic issue which arises in genetic screening revolves about the personal meaning of being labeled genetically aberrant. It is nearly impossible to make statements about the personal significance of being marked genetically deviant outside of some very general observations. Perhaps the most immediate significance of such knowledge for a person revolves about its impact on his conception of himself as a complete person and the interpersonal and social derivatives of this self-conception. Within the latter we are concerned in pursuing the possible impact on conceptions of marriageability and parenthood.

Genetic screening may hold significantly different social and psychologic meaning for a person, depending on when in his reproductive career the knowledge is acquired. If screening is conducted prior to marriage it may bring about changes in (1) a person's desire to get married, (2) his choice as to an acceptable mate, and (3) his desire for children. If, on the other hand, carrier status is disclosed within an established family unit, husband and wife may experience severe and chronic dissatisfaction with each other as reproductive partners and possibly seek other mates.

The disclosure of carrier status may entail the adoption of a negative evaluation of the self, especially when emphasis is on the aberrant condition and no weight is given to the "normal" characteristics of a person. This appears to be the case, since the disclosure of carrier status and the transmission of information in clinical genetics seems to be primarily on emphasizing disease and disorder – with little attention given to limiting the significance of such emphasis or to emphasizing that outside of carrying a specific disorder an individual is "normal."[18] This would appear to be especially true in nonmedical screening programs where individuals are provided with information relative to their carrier status and there is little professional information provided about the significance of this information or what such information may mean for the individual, not just at his current age but in the future as well. In such situations the status of a carrier may become so potent as to eclipse the normal aspects of the person to such a degree that the individual no longer sees himself as capable of entering into and meeting such usual social activities as marriage. The scientific label of genetic disease carrier could acquire a psychologic interpretation for the person which could threaten his sense of personal worth and integrity. In turn, changes in one's sense of personal worth can alter the degree to which an individual feels sufficiently competent to acquire and execute such social roles as mate and parent.

It is also possible that, if genetic screening is performed prior to marriage, the information as to one's genetic or chromosomal health may become explicit premises guiding the mate selection process. Available data suggest that the seeking of information about one's genetic health prior to marriage is quite unusual at the present time; genetic counselors report that only 7% of the individuals they counsel seek such counseling prior to marriage.[19] In the majority of these cases, individuals know they are related and are interested in the consequences of their common ancestry. If disclosure of carrier status does not remove the individual from the marriage marketplace, it may significantly affect routine mating patterns, making for assortative mating not only on the basis of phenotypic characteristics but also on gene or chromosome type. Heretofore, poor health has significantly affected a person's chances of marrying, but this reduction in chances occurred mostly at the extremes of severely disabling phenotypic disorders.[20] Just as individuals with certain mental and physical characteristics are preferred as mates today, different carrier statuses may take on degrees of preference in the future. As such, individuals with specific genotypes could become preferred mates, and those with other genotypes could become less desirable. The development of such preferred genotypes does not seem completely beyond possibility in a culture where there is a strong emphasis on getting ahead and being the best. This would seem to be especially true when it comes to parental considerations as to children, and parental desire for children to have as many opportunities as possible to advance in life. A threat of severe or even a mildly disabling disease would seem to cast serious doubt on parental capacity to provide their children with the best possible opportunities and hence cast doubt on the person identified as a carrier as to his desirability as a mate.

Disclosure of carrier status may thus most significantly affect an individual's desire for parenthood. It is probably in the role of parent that the repercussions of carrier status are most immediate and most likely to alter life expectations and experiences. Reproduction remains an important goal of most marriages. Factors which lessen the chances that an individual can competently meet this role of parent operate to reduce the desirability of such a person as a spouse. Personal worth and problems of inferiority complexes are major issues confronting those afflicted with overt phenotypic diseases.[21] It is certainly the case that parents who today experience the birth of an afflicted child feel considerable anguish and experience changes in their self-conceptions. In a study of parents of children affected with Down syndrome, Antley and Hartlage found that these parents exhibited considerably higher levels of anxiety, hostility and depression than did a group of controls.[22] Likewise, Birenbaum, in his research on parents of abnormal children, has noted the social and psychologic problems and adjustments which such parents go through in adapting to their unexpected situation.[23]

While our own understanding of genetics has shifted from the realm of animism to naturalism, and the change in our view of genetics from social problems to medical issues has greatly reduced the chances that individuals will interpret carrier status as a sign of personal worth, this remains something of a problem. The realization that one has a genetic anomaly may acquire the status of a severe personal problem if individuals interpret nature's machinations as punishment resulting from their own conduct. In a culture which stresses individual initiative and contains elements of a moral code which subscribes to the notion of cosmic justice, or "as ye sow, so shall ye reap," it is not uncommon for individuals to attempt to translate misfortune from the realm of chance to that of personal responsibility.

Different subcultures in this society provide for variation in the probability of such interpretations occurring. As Zuk has noted in his studies of parental reactions to the birth of mentally abnormal children, the religious beliefs of some groups permit them to see personal problems in terms of a test of their moral strength.[24] Therefore, they are less disposed to interpret such an event as the result of personal conduct and more likely to see it as the trial of their faith. In these situations the psychologic repercussions of abnormality, genetic or otherwise, are likely to be less severe than when individuals attempt to see such situations as a mark of personal worth. Nevertheless, while scientific information may remove some of the misunderstanding about the actual mechanisms involved, it may not remove all of the doubt, suspicion and fear regarding one's own involvement in the etiology of becoming the bearer of genetic misfortune.

The significance of genetic screening in any of the above situations resides in part in the nature of the disorder the individual might transmit, as well as the cultural and social significance assigned to that particular disorder. As suggested, individuals with diabetes in their family or those carrying other noncosmetic genetic disorders may suffer relatively little social discrimination in this culture, while those at risk for producing a mentally abnormal child may experience much more severe and chronic social ostracism. Also, if a particular disease can be effectively treated and affected individuals can be expected to live relatively normal lives, or if prenatal diagnosis and selective abortion are available, then the repercussions of being a carrier may be reduced. However, the burden reduction in these situations may occur primarily in the area of the actual suffering of the affected and the financial and social burden an affected person might have brought to a family.

Fletcher, in a recent paper discussing the evolution of attitudes toward congenital abnormalities, has argued persuasively that the technology of applied genetics, especially the development of amniocentesis, may provide the basis for significant changes.[25] Humane values have provided for an indulgent attitude in the past in prevailing attitudes toward congenital abnormalities. He suggests, however, that with the availability of the technology and know-how permitting prevention of many genetically based congenital abnormalities, there may be developing as a corollary a social attitude which demands such use. In general, if a congenital abnormality can be avoided, then it should be, and those individuals who do not partake of these advances will be socially ostracized. If, in fact, such social attitudes toward technology utilization are developing, then individuals carrying genetic disorders will perhaps be under considerable pressure to avoid situations where they may risk having a child with a genetically based disorder. This could entail not marrying or significantly altering the individuals one would consider as acceptable mates.

The development of such an attitude seems possible, especially in light of an increasing societal concern with resources and the most effective and efficient utilization of those limited resources. Handicapped children, especially those that can provide no means of support, often become dependent on society. They can incur for the state significant financial burden and may come to occupy a significant proportion of available hospital and medical treatment facilities.[26,27] The burden such children impose could come to be viewed as oppressive by society, since these children could have been avoided in many cases. Those individuals who could avoid defective children by being informed of their carrier status but do not seek such information might come to be socially ostracized as malingerers in the use of medical technology, "deviants" for whom society has to pay the cost of their malingering.

Finally, it may be the case that the individuals who carry the diseases for which genetic screening has been developed first may incur much personal unhappiness and social ostracism because they are the first to be singled out and labeled as "unhealthy." Pursuing this argument, as it becomes possible to detect carrier status for a larger and larger number of diseases, the novelty of being a carrier and the problems in adapting to it may be lessened. Geneticists claim that almost all individuals carry between five and eight deleterious genes, which if paired with the appropriate gene will produce a high risk of disease abnormality in offspring. When carrier detection becomes possible for large numbers of diseases, then most people can be diagnosed as a carrier of something, and the psychologic and social burden of being so designated may be lessened.

This argument has some force. Two things need to be mentioned, however. First, while we all may carry deleterious genes, some of the resultant diseases will be more socially unacceptable than others; thus, carriers of these diseases will almost always incur more personal and social burden than those carrying less socially disapproved diseases. Second, it can not be forgotten that disclosure of carrier status will mean for many that they are, in one sense, unfit for parenthood. Whether one shares this unfitness with many or only a few, it can still serve as a mark of being not necessarily different, but of being somehow unhealthy. As long as parenthood remains a popular status in this society, carrier status disclosure offers an opportunity for anxiety and feelings of lack of self-esteem.[22]

Genetic Screening and the Family

While the first and perhaps most significant impact of being labeled a carrier of a genetic anomaly may affect feelings of self-identity and self-worth, such feelings can have a pronounced effect not only on an individual's contracting a marriage but also on his maintaining a satisfying marriage relationship. It is in the roles of spouse and parent that disclosure of carrier status may most significantly alter an individual's social relationships. In order to more fully appreciate the potential impact and risks of carrier status disclosure, it will be beneficial to comment briefly on marriage and parenthood.

Marriage remains one of the basic institutions of society, and within marriage, reproduction remains one of the primary functions of the family. Even though there is considerable social pressure to reduce the size of families, as witnessed by such movements as Zero Population Growth, it is important to note that it probably still is as important as ever that a family be both a social and biologic entity in our culture. While birth rates are dropping and the rate of population increase is decelerating, it remains a fact that a larger proportion of couples are having at least one child than ever before in the history of this nation.[28] While it is less important that one be a parent several times, it is still important that one be a parent.

There are several things worth noting about marriage and reproduction in our postindustrial society. It has been argued that with the shrinking size of the American family, there may be an attendant increase in the desire that any child a couple has to be as perfect as possible. The realization that one's genetic constitution is abnormal poses a threat to fulfilling this desire. It is also reasonable that, as the social functions for the family decrease from broad, multitudinous activities to those centered largely about the satisfaction of the adult members, the meaning and significance of children as ego extensions of the parents may be increasing. In these circumstances realization that one carries a genetic problem and risks a defective child can be perhaps more devastating than it was earlier, when a family could have many children and when children were desired for more reasons than self-expression.

With the importance of marriage and reproduction in this culture, in terms of both societal normalcy and individual fulfillment, the advent of genetic screening may convey much personal unhappiness and pose some new barriers to many individuals who want to maintain a satisfactory marriage relationship. If the disclosure of carrier status occurs within established family units there are risks that the individuals involved may find their marital life seriously compromised; in fact, such disclosure may lead to marital discord and even dissolution. While there is no information on the effects of carrier status disclosure in screening programs on established marriages, such disclosures do occur within routine genetic counseling. Stevenson et al in England recommend not disclosing full information in genetic counseling unless there are overriding considerations.[29] They see potentially serious harm to established marital units by informing the couple as to the specific locus of genetic responsibility when the couple either already have or are facing a significant risk for a diseased child. They argue that it is better to simply inform the the parents that their child has a genetic defect and that both parents contributed to the genetic make-up of the child. Via this procedure counselors feel they can effectively diffuse feelings of responsibility that may develop on the part of one parent with the birth of a genetically defective child and thus avoid potentially serious marital discord. Certainly there can be severe feelings of remorse and responsibility concerning the birth of an afflicted child.[22] Studies by Agle on mothers of hemophilic children suggest that such mothers very often experience severe guilt feelings.[30] It is not uncommon for these mothers to overreact to the condition of their sons, at times making such children either recluses or exposing them to significant risks by encouraging reckless behavior. Chronic feelings of guilt and remorse have become problems that a number of doctors have commented on with regard to parents of defective children. The diffusion of responsibility in cases where one parent is in essence genetically responsible incurs a host of problems concerning full disclosure of information and other ethical issues which the doctor must consider in light of the potential psychologic disturbance that carrier status identification may induce. Carter et al in a longitudinal study of genetic counseling couples in England, provide some additional comment on the possible effects of carrier status disclosure.[31] Their data show that for individuals who had gone through counseling and presumably been informed as to the nature of the genetic mechanisms involved, the rate of marriage dissolution was no greater than for the comparable age cohort in England at that time. However, if one recomputes the Carter data, arraying it so that a comparison is made between those who reported that counseling affected their reproductive expectations and those who said that it did not, the rate of divorce in the former group is nearly three times the national average while that for the latter group is below statistical normalcy for the specific age cohort. These admittedly limited data suggest the pronounced impact that carrier status detection may have on married couples, especially on those who perhaps have not completed their reproductive careers. Not only can disclosure of carrier status bring about changes in reproductive plans but, as the Carter data suggest, it may bring about changes in reproductive partners. These data reflect the value and importance that individuals still place on reproduction and on their intense desires to produce normal children. While genetic screening and carrier disclosure may not pose such problems in situations where a couple have already completed their reproductive career or where such procedures as amniocentesis are possible, if such options are not available there can be significant risk to carrier individuals in terms of maintaining a stable and satisfactory marital unit.

It is worth noting also that while genetic screening may expose the recurrence risk that a couple face in reproducing, the development of medically effective and safe procedures for artificial insemination donor has opened a route by which known carriers of genetic defects, in some situations, can have children and not risk a diseased child. Couples who opt for artificial insemination donor can, of course, achieve the status of social parents. But in the process one of the partners is removed from the role of biologic parenthood. What results is the construction of a socially constituted family, with biologic parenthood limited to only one member. Such a situation is at variance with the culturally prescribed social and biologic integrity of the family. While this situation may be acceptable to some, as Carter and others have noted in England, artificial insemination donor is generally unacceptable to genetic counseling clients.[31]

Within the American culture there is also considerable documented resistance to utilization of artificial insemination donor. Francoeur reports the results of a recent national survey polling Americans on their attitudes toward artificial insemination.[32] This study found that on the average no more than 26% of the individuals approved of artificial insemination donor and only a slight majority, 55%, approved of artificial insemination husband. Sexual exclusiveness and natural parenthood remain strong personal desires of many if not most; thus the social and biologic integrity of the family is an important constraint limiting widespread acceptance of such procedures as artificial insemination donor. With this option closed for many, and with the option of adoption rapidly closing, the disclosure of carrier status may take on more and more psychologic significance for individuals desiring marriage and parenthood.

Summary

In this paper we have attempted to explore some of the social and psychologic issues that may be involved in genetic screening. In particular our attention has been given to discussing carrier status as a health issue, and to reviewing the impact carrier status disclosure may have on an individual's physical, psychologic and social functioning.

Noting that there appear to be few, if any, physical signs or illnesses associated with carrier status, the brunt of our attention was turned to the possible psychologic and social disabilities which may occur. Our attention has focused on how identification as a carrier of a genetic disorder may alter an individual's self-concept, and how such changes in turn may alter his ability to maintain or establish "routine" social relationships in this culture. In general, it appears that there is the potential in genetic screening and concomitant carrier status disclosure for considerable alteration of routine social relationships, and as a corollary the advent of this new biomedical technology should be made with such possibilities in mind. Of necessity our discussion has been limited, and there are undoubtedly many more aspects to genetic screening than those mentioned here. For example, there is already much interest in the possible impact of carrier identification on employability.[9]

A full consideration of such issues should accompany the scientific development of our ability to designate each other as bearers of "normalities and abnormalities." The medical profession has known for some time that individuals who suffer from severe disease often exhibit a stereotypic sequence of stages that they go through in adapting to their situation. There is often denial, rejection, severe depression and, finally, some type of adaptation. Any event that a person experiences which causes significant alterations in his life expectations is likely to give rise to such a sequence of psychologic adjustments. Certainly, learning that one is the carrier of a genetic disease and that one may pass it on to one's children can be such an event. As we have discussed, it is an event which may call for changes in marriage plans, mates and parent expectations. Some may consider these as good and others may not. Regardless, the public as well as the professionals involved in genetic screening should be aware of these possibilities and view genetic screening in light of its possible sociopsychologic effects.

The meaning attached to carrier status disclosure differs significantly from person to person. While many would readily welcome such information because it might enable them to avoid having a defective child, others would not want such information, fearing what it might mean about them or their spouses, their integrity as individuals and their fitness as parents. Effective and efficient utilization of genetic screening requires that both the public and the medical profession be aware of this variation and the issues which carrier status identification may entail. Genetic screening programs must include, along with provisions to assist individuals in using the information gained through screening to avoid illness and disease, provisions which enable them to learn to live with the personal knowledge that the new genetics provides about themselves and others.

References

1. Haller, M.: *Eugenics.* New Brunswick:Rutgers University Press, 1963.
2. Ludmerer, K.: *Genetics and American Society.* Baltimore:Johns Hopkins University Press, 1972.
3. Albrecht, J. and Day, N.: *A Survey of Genetic Counseling Facilities in Massachusetts.* (Supplementary survey of physicians and genetic services which they provide.) Massachusetts Department of Public Health, 1971.
4. Harris, M. (ed.): *Early Diagnosis of Human Genetic Defects.* Washington: Government Printing Office, 1971. H. E. W. Publication No. (NIH) 72-75.
5. Sarason, S. and Doris, J.: *Psychological Problems in Mental Deficiency,* 4th ed., New York:Harper and Row, 1969.
6. Stevenson, R. E. and Howell, R. R.: Some medical and social aspects of the treatment for genetic-metabolic disease. *Ann. Amer. Acad. Polit. Social Sci.,* pp. 30-37, Dec. 1972.
7. Osborn, F.: *The Future of Human Heredity.* New York:Weybright and Talley, 1968.
8. Gottesman, I. I. and Erlenmeyer-Kimling, L.: Prologue: A foundation for informed eugenics *Social Biol.,* suppl. 18, pp. 51-58, Sept. 1971.
9. Frankel, M.: *Genetic Technology: Promises and Problems.* Washington:George Washington University, 1973.
10. Parsons, T.: *The Social System.* New York:The Free Press of Glencoe, 1951.
11. Wilson, R.: *The Sociology of Health.* New York:Random House, 1972.
12. Coe, R.: *Sociology of Medicine.* New York:McGraw-Hill Book Co., 1970.
13. Scott, R.: *The Making of Blind Men.* New York:Russell Sage Foundation, 1969.
14. Kassebaum, G. and Baumann, B.: Dimensions of the sick role in chronic illness. *J. Health Social Behav., 6*:16-27, (Spring) 1965.
15. Tringo, J.: The hierarchy of preference toward disability groups. *J. Spec. Ed., 4*:3:295-306, 1970.
16. Harasymiw, S.: Prejudice toward minority groups and familiarity with disabilities: Their relationship to attitudes toward the disabled. Unpublished manuscript, New England Special Education Instructional Material Center, Boston University, 1971.
17. Jones, S. R., Binder, R. and Donowho, E.: Sudden death in sickle-cell trait. *New Eng. J. Med., 282* (suppl. 6):323, 1970.
18. Scheinfeld, A.: The public and human genetics. *Acta Genet. Statist. Med.,* 7:487-492, 1957.
19. Sorenson, J.: *Applied Human Genetics Study: Final Report.* Princeton:Princeton University, 1971.
20. Slater, E., Hare, E. and Price, J.: Marriage and fertility of psychiatric patients compared with national data. *Social Biol.,* suppl. 18, pp. 560-573, Sept. 1971.

21. Geis, H.: The problem of personal worth in the physically disabled patient. *Rehab. Lit., 33*:2:34-39, 1972.
22. Antley, R. and Hartlage, L.: Psychological responses to genetic counseling for Down's syndrome. Unpublished manuscript, Indiana University School of Medicine, 1973.
23. Birenbaum, A.: On managing a courtesy stigma. *J. Health Social Behav., 11*:3:196-206, 1970.
24. Zuk, G. H.: Religious factor and role of guilt in parental acceptance of the retarded child. *Amer. J. Ment. Defic., 64*:1:139-147, 1959.
25. Fletcher, J.: Attitudes toward the defective newborn. Unpublished manuscript, July, 1973.
26. Danes, B.: Genetic Counseling, *Med. World News,* pp. 35-41. Nov. 6, 1970.
27. Stevenson, A.: The load of hereditary defects in human populations. *Radiat. Res.,* suppl. 1, pp. 306-325, 1959.
28. Freedman, R., Whelpton, P and Cambell, A.: *Family Planning, Sterility, and Population Growth.* New York:McGraw-Hill Book Co., 1959.
29. Stevenson, A. C., Davison, B. and Oakes, M.: *Genetic Counseling.* Philadelphia:J. B. Lippincott Co., 1970.
30. Agle, D. P.: Psychiatric studies of patients with hemophilia and related states. *Arch. Intern. Med., 114*:76-82, 1964.
31. Carter, C., Evans, K., Roberts, J. and Buck, A.: Genetic clinic: A follow-up. *Lancet,* pp.281-285. Feb. 6, 1971.
32. Francoeur, R.: *Utopian Motherhood.* New York:Doubleday, 1970.

The Practitioner's View of the Values Involved in Genetic Screening and Counseling

Individual vs. Societal Imperatives

Robert F. Murray, Jr., M.D., M.S.

In order to better understand the practitioner's view of the values involved in genetic screening it might be helpful to define the term practitioner – before discussing the current concepts of screening and counseling.

What is a Practitioner?

A practitioner is defined as one who exercises an art, science or profession (as law, medicine or engineering).[1] The root of this term (practitian) is an alternative form of the word practition designating one acquainted or skilled by practice: a practiced or practical person.[1] In one sense, then, the practitioner, medical or otherwise, not only exercises his profession but must do so in *practical* terms. Beginning with Hippocrates and continuing to the present, this has meant an emphasis on those maneuvers the physician could carry out to improve the physical or mental condition of the patient. The practice or practical application of the medical art has taken place in the context of the doctor-patient relationship, which is governed by at least two rules: first, that confidentiality must be maintained; and second, that the practitioner must not knowingly harm the patient while trying to help him.

Most of the time the practitioner focuses attention on one person at a time. Any action taken is governed by the needs of the individual patient being dealt with at a given moment. Not only is the practitioner bound by

---

Robert F. Murray, Jr., M.D., M.S., *Associate Professor, Pediatrics and Medicine; Chief, Medical Genetics Unit, Howard University College of Medicine, Washington, D.C.*

the Hippocratic Oath and the generally accepted code of medical ethics to this course of action, but there are legal obligations promulgated by society which cannot be safely ignored. The basic nature and orientation of the medical practitioner, then, requires that he (or she) focus his skills on each individual patient in a practical, positive fashion, and both legal and moral pressures reinforce this orientation.

There has been a significant movement in modern medicine to widen the purview of the practitioner to include the family and even the community. The establishment of new departments of family practice and community medicine in medical schools reflects this growing trend. It is one thing to discuss and theorize about family and community health, but quite another thing to treat a family or a community for illness or to attempt to prevent illness on a large scale. The family and the community are, after all, collections of individuals who in the final analysis must be evaluated one by one. One may discuss the statistical alternatives of groups of people, but the outcome of a particular course of action for a given individual is either yes or no! Screening for genetically determined disease is one manifestation of the trend toward family and community orientation in modern medicine. This trend has been relatively recently thrust upon the medical scene in a climate where, heretofore, primary emphasis has been placed on the needs of the individual. Not only is the practitioner required to scan the family and also the community for the presence of diseased individuals, but this must be done in the context of a social climate where there is ignorance, confusion and fear regarding genetically determined diseases. The nature of these diseases is not understood by the layman and is often poorly understood by the practicing physician, because most practitioners have had little or no exposure to the principles that govern the genetic transmission and expression of these conditions.

From my perspective, then, the practitioner will often view genetic screening from the point of view of one who is:

1. Pragmatic in orientation.
2. Primarily concerned for the individual.
3. Oriented toward being able to do something for the patient.
4. Paternalistic and directive.
5. Weak in his understanding of genetics and genetic mechanisms.
6. Aware of, but not really oriented toward family or community medicine.
7. Really just beginning to accept the concepts of preventive medicine and what they mean.

With this overview of the practitioner and the climate in which he works, we should next establish some concept of genetic screening.

Screening in the Medical Setting

In the usual medical sense, screening has been defined as "the presumptive identification of unrecognized disease or defect by the application of tests, examinations or other procedures which can be applied rapidly." Screening tests sort out apparently well persons who probably have a disease from those who probably do not. (See paper by Lappé and Roblin in this series for an elaboration of this view.) A screening test is not intended to be diagnostic. Persons with positive or suspicious findings must be referred to their physicians for definitive diagnosis and necessary treatment.[2]

This definition encompasses the processes that practicing physicians generally agree are involved in screening. The presumption is that the person detected who is positive has a disease in some stage of development. It may be preclinical, early, moderate or late in its expression. Using this definition the asymptomatic carrier of a mutant gene who is identified in a screening survey, eg the person with sickle cell trait, might be classified as mildly affected. This was indeed the case in early classifications of sickle cell disease when only the sickling test was available for screening. Persons with sickle cell trait were diagnosed as having "sickling without anemia" or a mild form of sickle cell anemia. The essence of screening in the practical medical sense has been summed up by the phrase "early disease detection."[3]

In my view, the concept of screening ought to be broadened and modified if diseases with major recessive genetic determinants (eg Tay-Sachs disease or sickle cell anemia) are to be properly included. The definition of screening previously quoted should be modified to state that *genetic screening is the presumptive identification of unrecognized diseases, defects or healthy heterozygous carriers of mutant genes which may produce children with disease under appropriate circumstances, but which do not produce significant clinical disease in the heterozygous individual.* Genetic screening can be done by performing *reliable* and *accurate* tests, examinations or other procedures which can be rapidly applied.

In 1967, the WHO Scientific Group on Screening for Inborn Errors of Metabolism[4] reviewed the available literature "to consider whether and how screening programs for such disorders could improve the health of mankind." The committee felt that three criteria should be met before a genetic screening program could be unquestionably accepted:

1. Facilities for the validation of the presumptive diagnosis produced by the screening test should be provided.
2. The disorder being tested for ought to be amenable to treatment.
3. The socioeconomic effects of screening programs should be studied and taken into account in the deliberations that precede the institution of the program.

Another WHO scientific group met in 1971 to consider the problem of Genetic Disorders: Prevention, Treatment and Rehabilitation. In their view the obvious objective of screening was "to improve the quality of life for individuals and society as a whole by permitting the control of disease in affected persons."[5] The objective of genetic screening, they pointed out, is to detect the trait early enough to prevent harmful expression of the mutant allele. This can be done by prenatal detection followed by therapeutic abortion (eg Tay-Sachs disease) or by early postnatal detection of affected infants with early institution of treatment, as with phenylketonuria (PKU).

This committee also considered in depth the potential benefits of screening for the heterozygous carrier. They pointed out the possibility of reducing the frequency of diseased offspring by providing effective genetic counseling to heterozygous individuals who may use the information in mate selection or who may abstain from childbearing or choose another reproductive option should they marry another heterozygous carrier. But whether prevention of the recurrence of a genetic disorder is desirable, or the method chosen to prevent its recurrence is satisfactory, is a function of its recurrence rate and severity, as well as the attitudes and cultural mores of the couple involved which may be a consequence of the customs and laws of their society.

Screening, as it relates to genetic disorders, has introduced a somewhat new and unfamiliar dimension to the practitioner. It provides him with the potential for preventing disease in a manner not generally followed heretofore on a significant scale in modern medical practice; namely, the prevention of the birth or even the conception of genetically affected individuals. This is a change in position for the practitioner, for in the past when a life has been taken, it has been for the purpose of saving another life. (See articles by Powledge, Lappé and Roblin in this series for an expanded treatment of this topic.)

Not only must the medical practitioner expand his concept of screening and the indications for and consequences of it, but the concept of the nature of the individual manifesting in a detectable way an "abnormal" character must be modified. Rather than considering him (or her) abnormal, it must be understood that this is the natural state of affairs for the healthy heterozygous carrier of a genetically determined disease. The average practitioner does not understand, or has not incorporated into his thinking, the concept that all human beings are carriers of mutant genes and that we are now able to detect only a few of them. Furthermore, practitioners generally do not recognize that screening for genetic disorders will be an even larger and more important part of medical practice as the technology for this kind of testing is improved!

Genetic Counseling and the Practitioner

The definition of genetic counseling has undergone considerable evolution during the past decade. Fraser[6] recently defined the process of genetic counseling by listing the steps to be followed by the counselor:

1. Establishing the risk of recurrence of disease.
2. Interpreting this risk in meaningful terms.
3. Aiding the counselee to weigh the risk.
4. Reinforcing the risk and estimating its effect on the counselee through follow-up counseling.

This limited concept of the genetic counseling process has been broadened by Sly,[7] who defined genetic counseling as "the delivery of professional advice concerning the magnitude of, the implication of, and the alternatives for dealing with the risk of occurrence of a hereditary disorder within a family." But this concept is still too limited; a more comprehensive definition would include the clear communication of all the medical, social and genetic facts related to the condition under consideration, including the prognosis for the condition as well as the possible consequences of one or another mode of action. Counseling is an educational process and should provide emotional support, but should not be directive in the decision-making process of the counselee.

The modern practitioner may be aware of, but is often unfamiliar with the process and content of genetic counseling. He is not only often unaware of the way counseling is best done, but he is unfamiliar with the process and content of the usual counseling session. The physician is particularly unfamiliar with the idea that the patient to be counseled, in contrast to the usual situation with patients, should *not* be given advice. To make matters worse, the person to be counseled, all too often, expects that the physician will fill his traditional role and give direct advice about what he ought to do.

Not only are there significant differences in the time and content of genetic counseling from the usual doctor-patient relationship, but there are special problems involved in the communication of the concepts of the gene, its mode of inheritance and how it operates. On top of this, there is the extremely difficult task of getting across the idea of statistical recurrence risk, even when one is skilled in counseling.[8]

The practitioner is likely to see genetic counseling as inefficient, frustrating and confusing because its concepts and operation differ so sharply from the usual way he relates to patients. Thus, the practitioner is likely to view genetic screening and counseling as useful, but unfamiliar and in some instances as impractical adjuncts to medical care which he is obligated to administer so as to enhance the health and well-being of his patient, and under particular circumstances, of the family and the wider community. These modalities must be considered in the context of the traditional medical model, despite the inherent difficulties, since a drastic change in the practitioner's attitudes and patterns of thinking is unlikely to occur in the near future.

If the previously described view of the practitioner and the concept of genetic screening and counseling can be accepted for the moment as valid, it is now possible to examine the values related to and implicit in these processes which are so new on the medical scene.

The Values Held by the Practitioner

If one were to poll the medical community, it is unlikely that there would be unanimity of opinion regarding the most important values held by the practitioner, but certain ones would probably rank high on the list, including (1) survival, (2) well-being or happiness, (3) freedom, (4) knowledge or knowing, (5) truth-telling and (6) privacy or confidentiality.

Survival is the one essential value since the preservation of life is one of the prime reasons, if not the prime reason, for the existence of the medical profession. Without survival none of the other values would be significant. Screening programs which have as their goal early postnatal detection, followed by effective therapy, are readily understood and accepted. They fit quite well into the medical model. Screening at the prenatal level for chromosome defects or inborn errors of metabolism with the object of performing therapeutic abortion on the affected (or potentially affected) fetus would, on the surface, appear to conflict with this value. But there are other essential values that motivate the practitioner and which are supported by this kind of screening program. These are the companion values, well-being and happiness, which would be enhanced through the relief of the potential pain that would be experienced by the parents of an affected child, or that which might be experienced by the child affected by a condition causing deformity and pain even though the child's existence were limited. The happiness of the parents is further enhanced in this program because they can, with respect to the genetic condition in question, significantly improve their chance of having a healthy child.

There is another aspect of the value, survival; namely, the long-term survival of the species. The practitioner simply cannot, under the current contract that operates in the doctor-patient relationship, consider this value as a major factor in the decision-making process. To do so would conflict with the traditional obligation to do the best he can for the patient. He would also have to be directive in genetic counseling to achieve the objective of influencing reproduction among couples who are at risk to produce affected offspring. Moreover, carriers of mutant genes would have to be influenced to decrease their fertility or support a program of abortion of carriers. The number of abortions that would have to be performed on otherwise healthy babies is such to make this approach untenable.[9] From the medical perspective of one WHO scientific group there appears to be "no scientific or public justification for artificial prenatal selection against heterozygous carriers of recessive traits, even if reliable testing procedures can be devised for their detection."[5]

Both screening programs and genetic counseling operate to enhance the value of knowledge or knowing. This would be supported by the practitioner who, in general, believes it is better to know, especially when the knowledge offers parents "positive" options that will permit them to take practical steps to help themselves. However, some practitioners might raise questions about telling individuals of their carrier status for mutant genes before marriage particularly, because almost nothing is known about the effect of this knowledge on the psyche or self-image of the individual who is identified as being the carrier of a mutant or "bad" gene.[5]

Detection prior to marriage is not necessary where prenatal diagnosis is a practical option to couples at risk, as in the case of Tay-Sachs disease. (See the article by Kaback in this series.) In conditions which do not allow for this option, premarital screening becomes an essential maneuver so that mating can occur in a way that reproductive freedom will not be compromised more than for most other couples. This is the case with inherited conditions like sickle cell anemia and thalassemia or Cooley anemia where intrauterine diagnosis is not yet possible. In these instances there is the significant possibility of a sacrifice of social freedom since, for the carrier of sickle cell trait, about 1 in every 10 potential mates will be unsuitable if the individual wishes to avoid the risk of having an affected child.

There is also the question of the value of privacy for the carrier, particularly in light of traditional medical ethics which legally guarantees confidentiality. The unmarried heterozygous carrier might not wish to have his carrier status known since it might significantly compromise social mobility. There is already evidence that being a carrier of sickle cell trait can influence the status of the female as a suitable mate in rural Greek society.[10] The same may be true, although to a lesser extent, in the United States.

On the other hand, does the practitioner not have some obligation to inform other family members that they are at risk to be carriers, once he has discovered a member of the family who is heterozygous for a particular gene? A practitioner with the characteristics described earlier would only seek out other family members with the patient's permission if there is no clear course of action open to those family members at risk to be carriers. Moreover, they could probably get the information about their carrier status in the same way as did the practitioner's patient. On the other hand, if there is a viable option for couples at risk, and if seeking such an option, should they be at risk, would not cause them serious moral conflict, the practitioner would probably feel justified in choosing to violate the privacy and confidentiality of his patient in order to provide the values of knowledge and well-being to those genetically related to the patient, and therefore at risk to be carriers with the attendant risk for having affected children. Knowledge of genetic abnormalities, unlike that of other abnormalities, may not, in one sense, belong solely to the patient, because it has implications in the lives of his close genetic relatives (first-degree relatives) and to a lesser, but still significant extent for common conditions to the population at large.

Practitioners seldom have much ethical difficulty restricting the freedom of patients. They do it frequently when they prescribe dietary restrictions and medications or admit patients to hospital for diagnosis and treatment. Genetic screening obviously has the potential for introducing new kinds of restraints on freedom in mating and reproduction. The carrier who chooses knowledge may acquire with the information that he is the carrier of an autosomal recessive trait an implied restriction on his potential partners if he acts on the knowledge in what the practitioner might consider a sensible fashion. This means the carrier should act to avoid or minimize the risk for disease in his children. There need not be these restrictions if there is some effective method of treating affected children to prevent illness, or if there is intrauterine diagnosis for the condition in question and therapeutic abortion is acceptable; but these options are not yet available for conditions like sickle cell anemia, thalassemia major or cystic fibrosis. The carrier who plans to act on genetic screening advice may not only have mating options reduced, but may even find certain career opportunities restricted, or insurance premiums increased as in sickle cell trait. These policies have usually been instituted with inadequate justification.[11] By taking advantage of this option the carrier can avoid becoming part of that small population of couples where both are carriers of the sickle, thalassemia, hemoglobin C or other mutant beta chain genes, and thereby have a 25% risk of having a child with a hemoglobinopathy with each pregnancy.

From the practical standpoint of the practitioner, it would be better to follow the format of the Tay-Sachs screening programs instituted in various parts of the country. (See the article by Kaback in this series.) In this program, first the females and then the male spouses of those females found to be heterozygous carriers are tested. This provides an efficient method of identifying couples at risk which appeals to the practitioner. On the other hand, those couples identified may, after being counseled, experience restriction of reproductive freedom. If there is complete restriction there will be a significant lowering of the cases of affected children born, but even if reproductive restriction is only variably exercised, at least early detection of children at risk will be the outcome. Unfortunately, there is no significant clinical experience or conclusive evidence that guarantees that early detection and "prophylactic" therapy will have a significant effect on the number of crises or the longevity of the patient with sickle cell disease or thalassemia.

In my view, it doesn't really do patients a great deal of good to provide them with anxiety-provoking information that does not at the same time allow for some "therapeutic" course of action. Although the practitioner is interested in prevention of illness, his primary emphasis is still on treating the sick or disabled patient. He continues to be concerned for the living patient, and to shift his primary concern to the "potential" patient results in a kind of contradiction in thinking.

Is it *therapeutic* for the potential child, to counsel a couple at risk in such a way that they will avoid having their own biologic children? When a child with Tay-Sachs disease is aborted, is that "therapy" for the aborted child? In the context of the primary concerns of the practitioner, in both instances this must be considered therapy for the parents. Theirs is the suffering that will *definitely* occur and *theirs* is the well-being that will be preserved through knowledge of their potential for conceiving and giving birth to an affected child. They are really the patients who have come seeking treatment. So if the practitioner understands that he is really treating the potential parents for a genetically determined illness that *may* occur in one of their children, the partial sacrifice of their freedom and well-being may be justified because of the long-term benefit to them as parents.

If screening is carried out at the neonatal level and there is no known reliable way to prevent the progression or manifestation of illness, a conflict in values will again arise. The physician generally believes that if he knows about an illness prior to its clinical manifestation and also understands the natural history of the condition, he may be able to modify the clinical course of the condition. In the case of sickle cell anemia these conditions are partially satisfied since the condition can (with some difficulty) be diagnosed at birth, the natural history is at least partially understood and there is some information concerning the factors that may precipitate the recurrent acute episodes of pain called crises.[12] The major difficulty is that the clinical course of this disease cannot be predicted with accuracy for a given patient.[12] When the hemoglobin pattern consistent with the diagnosis of sickle cell anemia is detected at birth, there is no reliable way for the physician to say when and with what frequency a given patient will develop crises. Nor can one predict the severity of anemia or related problems merely by knowing that the patient has sickle cell anemia. The child with sickle cell anemia will usually have at least 6-12 months before anemia or other symptoms develop. But it may be years before the first significant sickle cell pain crisis occurs, although the first clinically significant vaso-occlusive crisis usually occurs by age 6. Is there really, then, a practical advantage in having the knowledge that the child has sickle cell anemia at birth? The answer is that we really don't know. The clinical value of prior knowledge of the presence of this condition for which there is no specific therapy must wait until well-designed studies have provided useful information. This question will become academic if and when effective treatment for sickle cell anemia becomes available.

It is in this kind of situation that the physician might choose to withhold information from parents whom he judges to be ill-prepared to handle information about the genetic status of their child and his potential illness. The physician would only reveal the diagnosis at the point when parents were prepared emotionally to accept the information without self-deprecation or reacting with excessive negativity or hostility toward the child. It is clear that the parents must have this information, but it would seem unjustified to disturb their sense of well-being with information at a time when they can do essentially nothing. If the physician has such knowledge, he can pass it along at an opportune time or make use of it if the child should have problems.

There is no doubt that the parents of a child with sickle cell anemia must be told at some time of their child's problem, but what of the parents of a child who has been found to have sickle cell trait during the same neonatal screening process? The present uncertainty about the potential for morbidity associated with sickle cell trait and the unconfirmed, anecdotal reports of sudden death in persons with sickle cell trait associated with severe exercise[13] and alcoholism[14] might have the effect of causing considerable anxiety, perhaps unnecessarily, in the parents. They can do nothing about the child's carrier status and, after all, the child is the one who may or may not act on his carrier status. The child, therefore, should be counseled. The practitioner might see some justification in withholding this kind of information from the parents because, in essence, they can only worry about it. But there is another aspect of this example: if the child with sickle cell trait is born to parents who have not been tested, there exists the distinct possibility that they both have the sickle cell trait and are at risk to give birth to a child with sickle cell disease. They would have to be informed of the child's status and its significance so that they might agree to be tested. In the majority of such cases, only one of the parents will be heterozygous for sickle cell trait; and only 1 in 12 couples so tested will be at risk for having children with sickle cell anemia. Is the anxiety that might be brought to the 11 couples by the early knowledge of a sickle-trait child worth the knowledge to the 1 couple not previously known to be at risk? If there were treatment or a definite alternative available, the practitioner might say yes, but with the current state of medical information the main basis for this approach would be to counsel the particular couple at risk so they might have the knowledge to make a reproductive decision appropriate to their life situation.

There is yet another aspect of this approach to screening that may occur with screening carried out at any time in childhood. This is the situation where nonpaternity is most likely to be detected; namely, the case where a child with sickle cell trait is found to have parents neither of whom has sickle cell trait. Such couples would be unusual but not rare, and the turmoil that might be brought into the family would mostly be unwarranted. This set of circumstances brought before the family in the guise of "helping" them is a veritable time bomb. If the situation is not skillfully handled, irreparable damage may occur to a family relationship that might otherwise have achieved some functional level of adjustment.

Obligations to the Individual vs. Obligations to Society and Future Generations

Over the past centuries the physician has focused his efforts on the concerns and needs of the individual patient; but as medical technology expands and becomes more sophisticated and, therefore, more costly, the practitioner feels increasing pressure to recognize the needs and concerns of the greater society. When such needs have been recognized in the past, especially with regard to preventive medicine, they have been focused on measures which, in the final analysis, would benefit the individual even though the initial effect might restrict one or more of the individual's values. The institution of regulations regarding sanitation or immunization against disease was designed to prevent illness in the individual, as well as to prevent the spread of communicable or infectious disease in a horizontal fashion throughout society.[3] (See the discussion by Green and Capron in this series for a contrasting view.)

The "new" emphasis on prevention of disease of genetic origin is on the prevention of the existence of persons who might have the potential for disease. To prevent disease in this context means preventing people. Societal concerns are pragmatic rather than humanistic. Representative of these concerns are the following:

1. What or how much do persons of a particular make-up contribute to the maintenance of social function and structure?
2. How much does it cost to maintain an "unhealthy" person as compared with the cost of preventing his birth or eliminating him?
3. How much of our limited economic and social resources, if any, can we afford to expend on this type of "unhealthy" individual?
4. How can the behavior of particular persons be altered or manipulated to ensure the survival of this society or social structure?

Individual rights and values get lost in providing the answers to these and other questions. Practitioners who become involved in their solution will tend to find themselves less and less concerned with the humanistic values that have supposedly motivated the practice of medicine since the time of Imhotep. Is the practitioner ignoring the societal imperatives to eliminate disease and save money?

It seems that he is doing just that with respect to the expenditure of large sums of money on patient-oriented therapy in the form of renal dialysis, kidney transplantation, cardiac transplantation and other very expensive medical-technologic solutions to chronic degenerative diseases. If the same funds were expended to institute early screening programs for kidney infection or factors that predispose to heart disease or even for large-scale educational programs, there might possibly be a much greater impact on the incidence of these and other diseases at considerably lower cost. In other words, practitioners are still primarily motivated by concern for the individual patient, and unless there are drastic changes in general philosophy they will continue to be. But this is only as it should be, since it is unlikely that any individual patient would be willing to have a medical decision made that was based on the needs of society rather than his or her personal needs. Patients who seek help in the setting of the medical model expect to be related to as individuals whose needs will come first in the mind of the practitioner.

Even though the needs and concerns of society cannot be minimized, society is, after all, a collection of individuals. Also, the purpose of genetic testing is ultimately to improve the health of mankind, but it would be inhumane to achieve this objective by destroying potentially sick children as is done in a veterinary sense or by manipulating the reproductive behavior of couples who are at risk for having affected children. Even if this approach to improving the health of society should be undertaken, there is no guarantee that the net effect would be improved health or even an improvement, in some measurable sense, in the gene pool. Medical selection against specific kinds of identifiable traits might have the long-term effect of selecting against other unknown genetic traits where the genes are linked to those being selected against. Our knowledge of the genetic composition and interaction of the genes in the human genome is so far from complete that to attempt to manipulate it or direct it in some haphazard way would either have no effect or possibly produce irreparable harm. It is difficult to justify inflicting emotional harm and anxiety on large numbers of people for the purpose of trying to effect a questionable change that might possibly, in the long run, be harmful. Although practitioners are aware of differences in the quality of human life, they have avoided making qualitative judgments on a larger scale about who should live and who should die. Where such judgments were involved they have left the decisions to those laymen whose own lives were intimately involved.

It is essential to this argument to realize that the "forward" march of technology will lead us to the point where virtually everyone will be identified as the carrier of some mutant gene, and considerably larger numbers of people will experience a compromise or limitation of rights and freedoms because of an emphasis on prevention that may evolve if current trends continue.

The practitioner must continue to juggle the values of the individual and the values of society, but it is probable that where these values come into conflict he will, as he has in the past, give preference to those humanistic values of the individual over those of society. The practitioner can feel confident in supporting genetic screening and counseling programs where individual rights and values are given first priority, because he does not have to compromise the ethical and moral values that have undergirded medical practice. At least, he knows that if he cannot help, he will do no harm. Some new kind of physician will have to be developed if the societal imperatives are to take first place. As a practitioner, I hope that this kind of physician will never be necessary or even desirable.

References

1. *Webster's Third International Dictionary,* 1966.
2. Commission on Chronic Illness: *Chronic Illness in the United States.* I. *Prevention of Chronic Illness.* Cambridge:Harvard University Press, 1957, p.45.
3. Wilson, J. M. G. and Jungner, G.: *Principles and Practice of Screening for Disease,* Public Health Papers No. 34. Geneva:World Health Organization, 1968, p. 13.
4. *Screening for Inborn Errors of Metabolism,* report of a WHO scientific group, Technical Reprint Series, no. 401. Geneva:World Health Organization, 1966.
5. *Genetic Disorders: Prevention, Treatment and Rehabilitation,* report of a WHO scientific group, Technical Reprint Series, no. 497. Geneva:World Health Organization, 1972.
6. Fraser, F. C.: Counseling in genetics: The intent and scope. In Bergsma, D. (ed.): *Genetic Counseling,* Birth Defects: Original Article Series, vol. VI, no. 1. Baltimore:Williams and Wilkins Co., for The National Foundation-March of Dimes, 1970, p. 7.
7. Sly, W. S.: What is genetic counseling? In Bergsma, D. (ed.): *Contemporary Genetic Counseling,* Birth Defects: Original Article Series, vol. IX, no. 4. White Plains:The National Foundation-March of Dimes, 1973, p. 5.
8. Leonard, C. O., Chase, G. A. and Childs, B.: Genetic counseling: A consumer's view. *New Eng. J. Med., 287*:433, 1972.
9. Motulsky, A. G., Fraser, G. R. and Felsenstein, J.: Public health and long-term genetic implications of intrauterine diagnosis and selective abortion. In Bergsma, D. (ed.): *Intrauterine Diagnosis,* Birth Defects: Original Article Series, vol. VII, no. 5. White Plains:The National Foundation-March of Dimes, 1971, p. 22.
10. Stamatoyannopolous, G.: Problems of screening and counseling in the hemoglobinopathies. In Motulsky, A. G. and Lenz, W. (eds.): *Birth Defects: Proceedings of 4th International Conference, Vienna, 1973.* Geneva:Excerpta Medica, 1974.

11. Bowman, J. E.: Mass screening programs for sickle cell hemoglobins: A sickle cell crisis. *JAMA, 222*:1650, 1972.
12. Powars, D. R., Lightbourne, R. E. and Benson, S. G.: A comprehensive approach to the care of the patient with sickle cell anemia. In Olafson, F. and Parker, A. W. (eds.): *Sickle Cell Anemia – The Neglected Disease.* Health Center Seminar Program Monograph Series, no. 5. Berkeley:University of California, 1973.
13. Jones, S. R., Binder, A. and Donowho, E. M., Jr.: Sudden death in sickle cell trait. *New Eng. J. Med., 282*:323, 1970.
14. Shope, E. S., Vodebruegge, C. F., Diggs, L. W. et al: Sudden death in unsuspected sickle cell disease. Presented at the Annual Meeting of the American Society of Clinical Pathologists, Boston, 1971.

Genetic Screening and Human Values

An Analysis

James M. Gustafson, Ph.D.

Introduction

Many arguments about ethical issues in medical care reflect basically different "moral visions," to use a term favored by Iris Murdoch.[1] This is the case also in discussions of genetic screening programs. For example, those who insist that genetic screening programs ought to be voluntary rather than compulsory are frequently weighted toward a concern for the maximum preservation of individual liberties. Their point of moral vision makes them sensitive to all encroachments upon the rights of persons to decide for themselves what medical knowledge about themselves they need, to determine whether they will bear children, and to have access to employment and insurance free from possible incrimination by misinterpreted medical information gained by compulsory procedures. In contrast, legislators and others who favor compulsory screening to detect carriers of certain genetic diseases are weighted toward what they presume will be benefits for both the individuals screened *and* for society. Their point of moral vision, for example, makes them sensitive to opportunities to act to avoid the births of children who may have the genetic disease being screened for, to avoid the potential economic and social costs that the births of children with certain diseases might incur, and to diminish what they judge to be avoidable anxiety and suffering for parents and for children.

When the moral visions of persons are in conflict with each other, it is not easy to overcome differences of opinion. This is so because preferences for certain values, certain moral beliefs and basic desires are at the roots of the differences, rather than errors in the logic of moral reasoning. The protagonist of compulsory screening tacitly or explicity *values* sufficiently

---

James M. Gustafson, Ph.D., *University Professor of Theological Ethics, University of Chicago, Ill.*

what he judges to be potential benefits to be willing to restrict the values of voluntary consent by individuals. He is willing to diminish the range of freedom of choice for citizens because he *believes* that under present circumstances other things are more important, that is, of greater value, than the measure of voluntary choice that would be lost. He *desires* to reduce anxiety, suffering and social and economic costs that are foreseeable and, given appropriate technologies, in part avoidable. While reasons can be given for what the person values, believes and desires, there are also affective qualities in valuing, believing and desiring which reflect his "vision," – his being weighted toward certain ends.

The conflicts of moral visions that can be identified with certain persons or groups often exist as tensions with the moral vision of individual persons. For example, a physician might be primarily oriented toward achieving a social policy which will reduce the incidence of particular genetic diseases in the national population, but be unwilling to say that to achieve that end it is permissible to impose compulsory genetic screening programs. He might believe that the policies which he favors ought also to take into account the liberty of individuals who are candidates for screening, and thus he would favor education and persuasion rather than legal compulsion as the means to bring persons and families to screening centers. The principal weight of his orientation is modified, or partially balanced, by the weight of other things he values, believes in and desires.

The purpose of this paper is to examine carefully what possibilities and what problems emerge when the primary language used to examine and justify genetic screening is one of *potential benefits.* I concur in the obvious assumption that if there were no benefits to be achieved there would be no point in screening. The practical outcome intended for the reader is to heighten his or her powers of discrimination in using the language of "benefits," so that opinions, judgments and decisions can be stated with greater refinement, clarity and self-critical awareness.

Other essays in this volume attend to the matter of voluntary vs. compulsory screening programs; for practical reasons it is prudent to assume a position on that issue here. We assume that the framework within which physicians and others work is one that minimizes the compulsory authorizations for screening. Much of what is written would be applicable as well to compulsory programs, but the intention is not to explore explicitly the issues within that type.

Two levels of decisions are involved in any discussion of human values as they arise in considerations of mass genetic screening programs. One is that of *general policies* with reference to the objectives or ends of screening. Policies cover classes of cases, and are designed to give general guidance to professional practice for the class of cases involved. The second is more *personal*; it is that of counsel given to particular individuals and the personal decisions they must make about their own choices and actions. I will try to indicate those points at which each level is primarily under consideration.

I have also sought to account for the particular ramifications and nuances of analysis that pertain to the different genetic diseases for which screening is now feasible, or might become feasible in the foreseeable future. By doing so, it is hoped that greater precision of analysis is achieved.

Benefits for Families

The primary stated purpose of the policies of most genetic screening programs is to benefit families. The principal benefit sought for families is the reduction of the number of occasions for severe human suffering* and for tragedy. This generalization is broad enough to cover all genetic screening programs, but cognizance must be taken of different genetic diseases and the screening that is appropriate to them.

The policy to screen newborns to detect the presence of treatable genetic diseases, such as phenylketonuria for example, has as its primary purpose the immediate institution of dietary treatment of the infant detected to have the disease. Such early detection and the proper reduction of phenylketonuria in the course of therapy benefit the primary patient by permitting him to avoid the normal sequence of mental retardation and hence to develop more normally.[2] The family benefits by having a healthier child, freed from some or all of the symptoms of an illness that would otherwise make his life more difficult physically, and perhaps emotionally and socially. In distinction from adult heterozygote screening programs, the purpose here is not to reduce suffering in the family by the prevention of births of diseased infants, but rather to proffer aid to an individual with genetic disease.

Screening programs for Tay-Sachs disease are examples of the former. The foremost purpose of such programs is to offer an opportunity for families to have children free of that fatal and untreatable disease. The obverse side is to provide the opportunity to avoid the anxiety, suffering and economic costs that having a Tay-Sachs child creates.

---

*A detailed analysis of the use of the term *suffering* follows in a subsequent portion of this paper. For the present its use is intentionally undifferentiated and vague.

The justification for a Tay-Sachs screening program can take the following more precise form. To give birth to and to care for a child with Tay-Sachs disease results in severe anguish and great economic costs to the family. Since there is at present no therapy, the child is destined to die at an early age. The parents are in a situation without hope for the child's life, and must cope with observing a child they love as he (or she) deteriorates through a course of many months. This anguish and cost are technically avoidable if certain conditions are met. The Tay-Sachs screening programs and the procedures that are available for follow-up in relevant instances establish these necessary and sufficient conditions.

If all adults of childbearing age in the high-risk population are screened (primarily Ashkenazi Jews of eastern European ancestry), then all matings between carriers of Tay-Sachs disease can be identified. Minor variations of this scheme, such as testing only married couples, are present in contemporary programs.[3] Genetic counseling of such couples is designed to make them aware that they have a 25% probability that each child they conceive will have the disease. If these couples either have no biologic children of their own, or if they employ artificial insemination with noncarrier donor semen, or if each pregnancy is monitored by amniocentesis and each fetus detected to have the disease is aborted, then it is possible for them to avoid bearing a Tay-Sachs infant. Thus far we have established the conditions necessary for personal decisions by the relevant couples.

A justification for a policy for screening large numbers of persons must take into account other considerations. For the purpose of simplifying the discussion, we will confine our attention to the benefit of avoiding mental anguish on the part of parents, without introducing factors of economic cost to them, and to other possible social benefits to present and future generations. Even with this simplification, the considerations remain complex, for a mass screening program might *ipso facto* create and intensify the anxieties of many persons. To make the strongest case, two assumptions have to be made which are difficult to establish fully. These are that the anguish of parents of a Tay-Sachs infant, and the anxiety of a person who is a carrier but mated with a noncarrier, and the anxieties that might be created in the population being screened (1) can be in some sense "weighed" and (2) can be compared. Granted these assumptions, the argument in favor of a Tay-Sachs mass screening program can be made as follows. If the severe mental anguish of the relatively small amount of potential Tay-Sachs parents "outweighs" the more general anxieties that might be created in the more numerous matings between a carrier and a noncarrier and the rather more diffuse anxieties that might be raised in the still larger susceptible population,* then it is more beneficial to screen for Tay-Sachs disease than not to screen. By this calculus the benefits to families in which both mates are carriers would have to exceed the cost of anxiety to other families. (More extensive analysis of suffering, anxiety and the calculation of benefits follows.)

Before turning to benefits for individuals and society, it is important to note that each specific genetic disease for which screening is now or will become possible requires a particular argument with reference to benefits, since the severity of suffering to be avoided is different for different diseases, and the frequencies of the diseases are different. Also, as therapy is developed for some diseases, this factor will have to be taken into account in the arguments.

If the frequency of disease were taken to be the exclusive criterion for determining whether a screening program is warranted, that is, if the number of families who might potentially benefit from the program were the major consideration, a certain order of priorities for developing feasible screening programs could be established. For example, since type II hyperlipoproteinemia is far more frequent (1/100 to 1/200 newborns with no ethnic factor) than Tay-Sachs disease (1/3,000 to 1/4,000 births among Ashkenazi Jews), on the criterion of frequency of the disease alone, more families would benefit from the establishment of feasible screening programs for it than for Tay-Sachs. Since sickle cell anemia is more frequent among U.S. blacks (approximately 1/500 births) than cystic fibrosis is among U.S. whites (1/2,200 births), on this criterion sickle cell screening would deserve the higher priority since proportionately more families potentially would benefit. However, we note that because of the disparity in size of the two populations, the actual number of families affected would be quite comparable. (In 1968, for example, we would have expected 1,062 black offspring with sickle cell anemia vs. 1,324 whites with cystic fibrosis [calculated from birth rates for 1968].)

No single criterion, however, is sufficient in itself to determine which diseases should be screened for. The severity of the disease also has to be taken into account. "Severity" is also ambiguous in some respects. If it refers to the person who has the disease, to be a meaningful criterion for comparative evaluations and justifications some way would have to be found to compare the severity of the suffering of a Tay-Sachs infant with that of a person with sickle cell anemia, and that of a person with cystic fibrosis (to confine the comparison to autosomal recessive conditions).

*The relative proportions of these groups is roughly 1:111:3,221 (assuming a gene frequency for Tay-Sachs disease of approximately 0.017, which is based on a homozygote frequency of 1 in 3,600 or a $q^2 = 0.00029$.)

Some meaningful criteria of comparison can be established, such as life expectancy and the degree of incapacitation of normal bodily functioning. If "severity" refers to the suffering of the family of the diseased person, some common criterion needs to be developed by which to compare the anguish of a family with a hemophiliac child with that of a family whose child might be detected (in the foreseeable future) to have Huntington chorea. When frequency is coupled with severity to determine what sorts of screening should be supported or what future screening should be developed for the sake of relieving the suffering of families, any argument in favor of one of the other programs becomes complex. An analysis of some of these complications follows in "Issues for More Precise Exploration."

How the suffering of families can be avoided by screening adds another issue. In Tay-Sachs screening the anguish is to be avoided by not bearing children with the disease; with amniocentesis and abortion available, a couple can be sure they have children without Tay-Sachs disease. In sickle cell screening and its follow-through procedures the options at present are not as simple: the disease is not fatal at an early age; the degree of incapacitation is not as great; prenatal detection is currently not possible, etc. Screening of newborns for the sake of detecting treatable diseases, as in the case of phenylketonuria, does not avoid anxiety in the way that the Tay-Sachs program can insure; yet the therapy does provide an alteration in the form that familial care and concern take.

Other essays in this series provide more detailed analysis of the differences between genetic diseases and the implications of these differences for the feasibility of particular types of screening programs. Here we are concerned only to call attention to the extensive variation in diseases in order to indicate what some of the implications of the differences are for how one would make an argument in various instances for programs of genetic screening on the basis that they enable families to benefit, particularly by avoiding or decreasing human suffering.

Benefits to Individuals

Screening programs are justified not only with reference to benefits for families, but also to specific individuals. One class of "individuals" is those whose birth is prevented, and thus for whom suffering is avoided. (This raises the larger question of whether one can define – for another – what is a life worth living.) Another class is newborn infants. The conditions under which they might benefit vary according to the diseases that can be tested for, and to the technologies available at a given time.

Screening for carrier state in parents makes possible the prediction of whether their infant will have the specific disease, or what the probability of risk is that an infant will be affected. The screening of parents provides them with information that can be taken into account in their decisions about procreation. For example, if both parents were detected to be carriers of sickle cell trait, and if they determined that the risk of bearing an affected child was in their view a "high" risk, and if they judged that a child with sickle cell disease would be severely incapacitated as it matured, they might choose not to procreate. Their choice would be defended on the grounds that having a child would be to inflict a probable risk of suffering on it, and thus for its sake (the "non-child") they will not reproduce. Given the greater severity (in terms of many years of suffering, constant pain and threat of death) of Huntington chorea and hemophilia, a parallel argument of greater cogency could be made by parents known to have a high risk for bearing children with these diseases. As medical science develops with reference to these diseases, the conditions under which greater precision of prediction can be made will occur. Thus it is conceivable that informed personal decisions can be made by parents which can avoid the possibility of persons being born who are destined to suffer from these diseases. Again, it may thus be for the sake of avoiding suffering that one refrains from giving birth to an individual whose incapacities can be predicted with a high degree of certitude.

The use of amniocentesis in pregnancies at risk for a Tay-Sachs infant is currently the most practicable follow-up from screening for carrier state in parents that can be defended on the grounds that it is more beneficial *to the child,* as well as to the family, that the affected fetus be aborted. The argument could be made in the following terms. The value of an infant's life is to be assessed not only in terms of its being the offspring of human parentage, and not only in terms of its survivability immediately at birth. Parents electing abortion may make a judgment for the sake of the infant that its normal development in its early months does not compensate in benefits to it for the inexorable course of deterioration that begins at approximately 6 months of age. Thus at least two criteria are implicitly or explicitly invoked to justify the abortion of the affected fetus: to have a meaningful and rewarding life requires the assurance of the longevity required to develop physical and mental capacities to a fuller extent than is possible in this case; and the satisfactions of normal development in the early months of the infant's life do not compensate for the extended deterioration of satisfaction that begins at 6 months. Thus it is beneficial to the fetus to be aborted.

These two criteria when applied to Huntington chorea (given the conditions of science and technology that would make procedures comparable to those used in Tay-Sachs programs possible) would be more ambiguous since the longevity is much greater, and since the period of life unaffected by the disease is much longer. The assessment of whether it is more beneficial for the individual not to be born will be more complex and less certain in its outcome. From this a general point comes to attention; namely, that benefits to individuals would differ potentially, depending upon which genetic disorder they had or carried. The precise substance of arguments will be different because of the specific situations and specific consequences that different diseases entail.

Screening has more certain benefits to individuals born where an effective therapy is available for the disease with which he is likely to be affected, or is known to be affected on the basis of newborn screening. Screening provides, in the former instance, a reliable basis for anticipating the likelihood that an infant is affected by a particular disease, and thus physicians are alerted to potential problems for which further testing might be required, and therapy used. In the instances of newborn screening for diseases, screening provides a correct diagnosis at an earlier stage for affected individuals, and thus eliminates possible diagnostic confusions, expenses, and delays in instituting therapy where it is available.

In distinction from the presumed benefits to a potential person by not being born, here we have specific therapeutic benefits to those who are born. The arguments to be made for screening in this class of cases are less complex and less ambiguous. Screening gives information which in turn makes possible interventions that are of immediate and long-range benefit to the child. Symptoms which will have debilitating effects on life can be controlled, and the possibilities for a normal development enhanced.

We have already noted how information from screening might benefit parents in making choices about procreation. More attention needs to be given to this and related matters. As tests continue to be developed that will increase the number of genetic defects for which persons can be screened, individuals will be able to have extended knowledge about their genetic make-up. This knowledge might be beneficial to them by increasing the amount of data that they would have accessible to make informed choices about selection of mating partner as well as about having children. The possible consequences of this are repugnant to some observers, but are anticipated by others for the possibilities provided for genetic responsibility. Whether they are repugnant or not reflects basic differences in value orientations.

Two questions emerge from this difference. First, when does the value of medical (in our case genetic) information about individuals reach a point of diminishing returns for them? No general answer to this question is possible because of the individual variables that must be considered. It is conceivable, for example, that a sure and certain knowledge that a person is neither a carrier of a gene for sickle cell trait, nor has the disease, can liberate a person from anxiety in circumstances such as now exist in the United States, namely, widespread information about the frequency of sickle cell among black persons. Knowledge that one is a carrier or has the disease, however, might produce anxieties, even under the conditions of adequate information about the defect. This is especially so with defects like sickle cell anemia for which there is no known cure and only ambiguous prospects for therapy at the present time.

As screening becomes more routine in conjunction with other medical tests, it is forseeable that a rather extensive genetic profile could be developed for many individuals. (See the paper by Lappé and Roblin in this volume.) The benefits they might achieve by having access to a genetic profile will be relative to a number of factors. One is their knowledge about and understanding of human genetics itself. Individuals will need to know about the severity of the defects of which they are carriers or which they have, they will need to know the frequency risks involved in having children, and they will need to know the genetic profile of their mates to assess those risks. Another factor is the availability of counseling facilities not only to provide an interpretation of the information but also to help individuals come to grips with any information that might affect their self-esteem, their desire for children and other deeply personal matters. A third factor is the availability of therapy for defects that are detected. No imagination is required to grasp the possibility that access to a genetic profile could create deep anxieties if the individual thereby gained information about serious defects for which there are limited therapies available.

If maximum genetic information about oneself is highly valued on the principle that information makes possible choices that are more rational, increase in the number of diseases screened for will be welcomed. If, however, it is judged that access to information without many other sustaining factors, including a high level of emotional maturity, might create undue anxieties and a sense of powerlessness (if no acceptable therapy is available), the circumstances are cloudier and more complex.

The second question that emerges is, where on a scale of value priorities does genetic health stand? For example, ought genetic information about oneself be incorporated into decisions to restrain social relations with a member of the opposite sex until there is certainty that mating will not issue in severely defective children? Or is the value of human love, and the spontaneity assumed in the language of "falling" in love, given higher priority than the value of possible freedom from a particular genetic disease for some offspring? These questions cannot be answered in the abstract, as the example of Dr. Michael Kaback's policies for Tay-Sachs screening help us to see.[3] (See the paper by Kaback et al in this series.) Kaback has articulated the view that only married persons of childbearing age ought to be screened for Tay-Sachs. Supporting this policy is the judgment that screening of adolescents, for example, might create in them a self-consciousness and anxiety about being a carrier that will be a detriment to the establishment of relationships in the freedom our society has traditionally valued. In this case, at the premarital stage the genetic health of potential offspring is lower in priority than the maintenance of a degree of spontaneity in establishing a relationship. But the status of medical technology makes such a decision easier in the case of Tay-Sachs. With the monitoring of pregnancies and with abortion possible, the birth of a Tay-Sachs infant can be avoided. In the instances of many other defects, however, prenatal diagnosis is not possible. Also, other diseases are not as severe.

Thus, the evidences and judgments which support Kaback's policy for postmarital Tay-Sachs screening do not necessarily support a similar policy for other genetic diseases. For example, it would not necessarily follow that a similar policy ought to be instituted for sickle cell screening. Since the disease in offspring is not as severe and is often not fatal (at least at an early age), the "genetic health" issue is of a lesser magnitude. Since sickle cell disease cannot at present be routinely diagnosed prenatally, the option of abortion of a diseased fetus is not generally available. Given these two conditions, it is plausible to argue that the genetic health factor ought not to be regarded at all in the mating of persons who carry the HbS gene. It is also plausible to argue that since the only "therapy" that is available to couples who are carriers is not to procreate, genetic information about carrier status of sickle cell is less beneficial to some couples than is ignorance about their status.

As science and technology progress, however, the conflict of values and the assessment of "costs" and "benefits" of information about the genetic profiles of individuals will increase and become more complex. It is already clear that information that individuals have about their "genetic profiles" is not necessarily beneficial in an unambiguous way.

Benefits to Particular Ethnic Groups

Since certain genetic diseases such as sickle cell anemia and Tay-Sachs disease have their highest frequency within identifiable ethnic groups, these groups bear a disproportionate burden of those illnesses relative to the society as a whole. Screening provides information that is necessary to reduce the incidence of such diseases and thus makes possible benefits for those ethnic groups.

Again, how the benefits will be achieved, and the probabilities of great success in the reduction of a disease, is relative to specific factors. As has been noted, the reduction of frequency of Tay-Sachs disease among Ashkenazi Jews is possible because of science and technology, which have developed the resources for testing carrier states and for prenatal testing. Also, the Jewish community in America can be readily organized and educated through its various institutions to participate in a program. The same technology is not available for sickle cell anemia; after carriers are identified there is no widely available prenatal test for the disease, and thus the choices available for reduction of the disease are different. Reduction of births by parents who are both carriers is the only sure way to reduce the frequency. Also, the black community is larger, the frequency of the disease is greater, and the task of mobilizing a program is probably more complex than in the Jewish community.

One of the benefits that public attention to sickle cell anemia might well develop for the black community is greater awareness of the overall health needs of its members. Until very recently this community has been virtually powerless to gain public support for its health needs, and such power as it has gained is still not sufficient to insure that these needs will be met. The aspiration of many persons concerned with sickle cell anemia is that attention to it will also have the consequences of wider support for other health problems.

The attention given to sickle cell anemia has led to a significant number of incidents in which individual blacks have borne the cost of actions based on mistaken judgments by employers and others. For example, on the basis of information that being at low oxygen partial pressures (as in surgical anesthesia) has been associated with deaths of blacks who are carriers of sickle cell trait, some airlines have dismissed black members of flight crews. The community as a whole has been subjected to potentially compulsory screening in several jurisdictions in America in a way that no other identifiable *ethnic group* has been isolated for such legal coercion. To judge the damaging consequences of this in terms of loss of self-esteem by some persons or of stigmatization of members of the group is not now possible. Yet there is some evidence that such consequences have followed.

A further possible deleterious effect on the black community might be pressure by the majority to reduce the number of births within this group. Since sickle cell anemia is an autosomal recessive condition there is a 25% probability of having an affected child when both parents are carriers. A policy of reducing the incidence of the disease implies justification of the elimination of potentially four births in order to prevent the birth of every one affected child. This can well be interpreted by an oppressed minority community to be a disguised justification for reduction of their birth rate. The difference between the technology possible for controlling Tay-Sachs and that for sickle cell anemia needs to be noted; the effectiveness of prenatal diagnosis in Tay-Sachs, with abortion of affected fetuses, does not pose the same threat to the Jewish community where compensatory reproduction is possible. Whereas an overall policy for both diseases might seek the reduction of the incidence of each in the relevant ethnic group, the personal decisions that parents must make to achieve that end are significantly different.

Benefits to Society

Three sorts of benefits to society can be invoked to support genetic screening. They are potential benefits to the health of the human race in future generations, the reduction of economic costs now required for caring for large numbers of persons with genetic diseases, and the diffuse aspiration that through screening programs large numbers of persons will learn basic information about human genetics.

The first is highly problematic for a number of reasons. The aspiration can be stated as follows. Genetic screening makes possible the identification of carriers and affected individuals of a number of genetic diseases. Given this information, and given possibilities for effective procedures to control births among those who would pass on the defective gene, it would be possible to reduce the frequency of severely deleterious genes in the human population. The society in view here includes the whole of the human race. The time span involved is indeterminate; if this objective is sought it would be supported on the basis of moral obligations each generation has for all future generations of the human species.

The unlikelihood of achieving such a global objective makes it highly problematic. The feasibility issue involves many factors. One question is whether under optimal conditions of genetic knowledge and optimal conditions of control of reproductive behavior a significant reduction of the frequency of at least certain diseases is possible at all. "Ought" implies "can," and whether this objective can be achieved is dependent upon complex factors of transmission of genes, beyond the scope of this paper.

This objective also raises serious questions in the light of the history of the earlier eugenics movement in the western world. That movement sought the elimination of certain "undesirable" strains in the population. Based on faulty science, it enshrined what are in retrospect unthoughtful and primitive laws requiring sterilization of certain classes of persons. Actions were sanctioned by such laws which not only infringed upon traditional individual rights and liberties but under totalitarian conditions led to the deaths of thousands of persons judged to be members of an undesirable class of persons. The invocation of this history serves as a warning for caution. The dramatic advances in the knowledge of human genetics are very recent and thus any policies considered now probably would be based upon more complete information. A series of judgments would be required about which genetic conditions ought to be the targets for future reduction. Who would have the authority to make these judgments? This question raises the questions of social power and potentially highly coercive social and legal measures. Assessment of the "costs" to other values held by human persons and by organized society in relation to the benefits to be achieved poses a most difficult problem; the defense of a highly interventionist eugenics policy would not be persuasive to large numbers of persons. If legal coercion were not used to determine who is restrained from bearing children, a severe degree of social pressure could still be exerted under a purported "voluntary" program.

These comments do not preclude the possibility of education of relevant persons about the possible consequences to future generations, or to the whole society of mankind, of their bearing children. Knowledge of human genetics creates the conditions under which the dimensions of responsibility are enlarged; present generations are "causally" responsible to some extent for the genetic health of future generations, and thus it can be argued that they also have a "moral" responsibility to them. The extensive temporal and social consequences of present actions in the realm of reproductive behavior are predictable to a higher degree of accuracy than in the past. Thus it is fitting to raise the consciousness of persons in this regard, and appropriate for them to take the consequences into account as they seek to discern the meaning of morally responsible parenthood.

The second foreseeable benefit to society is the possible reduction of public and private expenditures that are required to care for individuals afflicted with genetic diseases. The economic consequences of genetic diseases cannot be ignored simply because both family and public resources will always be scarce to a significant extent, and choices will always have to be made about what purposes are to govern their expenditures. Genetic screening is the first step in a series that creates the possibility of reducing the number of births of affected persons, and thus the possibility of reducing the amount of resources required for their care. (We shall not engage here in the required philosophic discussion of whether the reduction of economic costs involves in a strict sense a moral issue, and thus whether it can be argued that persons who have the capacity to relieve economic costs thereby have a moral obligation to do so.)

The pursuit of this social benefit is rich in ambiguities. It is demonstrably the case that genetic screening, when followed by courses of action that would reduce the number of births of defective offspring, makes possible the reduction of certain economic burdens to families and societies. This in itself, however, does not resolve the question of what human values *ought* to govern the allocation of resources. For example, ought legislators be more concerned to extend highway systems than to provide for health care for genetically defective persons? Ought families to be more concerned to have resources for luxuriant leisure than for the care of a defective child? Are the needs for national defense expenditures demonstrably more compelling than the needs of economically deprived families for public assistance and public institutional care for their genetically defective children?

Further, there is no political guarantee that resources saved by reducing the frequency of births of severely affected persons will be spent on measures that will increase the resources allocated for other health care. For example, it is not certain that expenses saved by reducing institutional facilities required to care for retarded children would be allocated to research which might reduce the costs involved to families, hospitals and other aspects of society in the care of persons who have hypertension. The intention to use genetic screening as a first step to reduce social costs will not necessarily lead to the allocation of those savings for social benefits of a medical sort.

The third social benefit of genetic screening is more diffuse, though its impact under some conditions might be more immediate than the first two. It is the benefit of a wider knowledge of human genetics, which in turn might affect family planning, public policy and other areas of human activity. Well-designed screening programs are highly educational and might have both circuitous and direct effects which are beneficial to society via the decisions individuals make regarding childbearing.

To have such social benefits the education that goes with screening must have certain qualities. Information that is not comprehended, or is misused, can create a great deal of anxiety and uncertainty. To have knowledge about human genetics without understanding the significance of the information for oneself, one's family, and for future progeny would lead to no great social benefits. Thus if screening is to have educational value, it must be accompanied by counseling that has as one of its purposes the communication to the persons screened of the arenas of human action and experience to which the knowledge is relevant. Indeed, apart from such education, the information might create anxieties which are detrimental, or might be misused by both the screenee and those who have genetic information about him.

Issues for More Precise Exploration

In the preceding portion of this paper, primary attention has been given to the actual and possible benefits of genetic screening programs. Some account has been taken of evidences which do or might qualify the beneficial consequences. The use of the term "benefits" has been intentionally rather imprecise; an effort was made to state certain claims in order to make clear in a general way what sorts of arguments could be made to support them.

An abundance of literature in moral philosophy exists from which much more careful analysis of the questions that emerge in using the language of benefits could be made. Some of the following questions are commonplace, but nonetheless remain important. When one is weighing various costs and benefits of screening programs, how does one quantify the qualities that are being compared? How does one quantify the essentially hypothetic avoidance of anxiety that not having a defective child makes possible? How does one weigh this against the psychic and social "costs" of having such a child? When economic benefits are invoked, how does one weigh these against the "value" of a human life that is not brought into being? Problems that are endemic to utilitarian ethics, and to a considerable extent in teleologic ethics (of which utilitarian ethics may be one form), have been commented upon in a vast amount of literature. It is not my purpose in this essay to render a philosophically sophisticated account of those issues, though noting their existence is prudent.

In the remainder of this paper, my intention is to develop three themes that emerge from the previous section. These are the use of "avoidance of, or relief from suffering" as a warrant for genetic screening and for the medical and personal decisions that might follow from it, the "special anxieties" that might result from genetic screening and the "false expectations" that screening might create both in parents and in society. References to particular genetic diseases are not as precise as they were in the previous section. Our assumption is that it is now worthwhile to look at these three themes more or less in their own right.

Avoidance of or Relief from Suffering

The suffering that genetic screening programs seeks to avoid is of three sorts. One is the physical pain and disability that are entailed in having certain diseases; the second is the mental anxiety and anguish that might be sustained both by having children affected by genetic diseases and by the children who are so affected; the third is economic suffering – the medical expenditures that reach proportions which require sacrifice by the family or the patient of their normal and customary standards of living. Screening and the counseling and medical interventions might follow at several junctures. To be screened and to avoid having children who might be affected is a choice for avoidance of suffering by not bearing children at all. To be screened, to have prenatal diagnosis and to abort affected fetuses is to make the choice of when fetal life is to be sacrificed for the sake of avoiding its suffering and the suffering of its parents and family. As I have shown, newborn screening provides the occasion for introducing therapy that limits the suffering both of the infant and of the parents who would have greater cares if the therapy was not available. Thus there are not only different sorts of suffering, but the avoidance of suffering takes place through different decisions relative to the diseases screened for and to the state of the arts involved in medical care. Not all the combinations of decisions will be articulated here; it is assumed that a more general discussion will permit the reader to see its pertinence to various instances.

Some discussion of the "status" of suffering is important. "To live is to suffer." This cliché is not without merit. Note that it is not "To live is *only* to suffer." It is not a statement from the point of view of an utterly pessimistic outlook on life. Rather, it recognizes that wherever there is physical life there is the possibility of pain; that human life is such that no persons are free from some measure of anxiety at least on some occasions in the course of their lives; that to be significantly related to others in the bonds of family and friendship involves care for one another (both in the sense of sustaining activity and in the sense of anxiety about each other); that bringing children into life involves economic costs which might entail inconvenience if not "pain" to parents and families. If these observations are correct, then the complete avoidance of suffering is beyond the bounds of human living.

Further, suffering under certain circumstances for certain persons is beneficial. The importance of physical pain as an indication of a disorder in the body is clear. Anxiety and anguish are sometimes intellectually and spiritually beneficial both for the person and for those to whom he is related directly or indirectly. Profound works of poetry and other literature, of art and of music have been affected by the anguish of their composers; the richness of human relations is sometimes enhanced by living through and sharing in the anxiety of other persons. Thus it cannot be affirmed that "suffering is evil" without significant qualification of the statement.

These remarks do not authorize the courting of suffering for the sake of its possible benefits; they do not make legitimate a strategy of suffering to enrich one's own life; they do not warrant the infliction of suffering on others for the sake of its potential usefulness to them. There is surely nothing morally or humanly wrong with avoiding suffering under the normal circumstances of human living. The line is sometimes very fine between the reprehensible avoidance of inconvenience and suffering for onself when one has *prima facie* duties and obligations to others on the one hand, and a pathologic courting of suffering for oneself by undertaking painful obligations to others on the other hand. Indeed, it is safe to presume that to avoid needless suffering is a legitimate rule of life. The problems in the application of such a rule of life come in the determination of what counts as "needless," or as "useless" (or other related adjectives). Somewhere between the two extremes of "suffering ought always to be avoided" and "suffering ought never to be avoided" lies a maxim that is difficult to state with precision, but is implicit as a base line in making decisions.

Thus far, what has been written suggests that the invocation of the avoidance of suffering as a warrant for genetic screening of various sorts, and for procedures which might follow from information gained through screening, is a very ambiguous claim to make. Yet, it is central to the human intention of all medical care. Our task now is to indicate some of the refinements that certain questions press upon the answerer.

First, is the suffering that could be avoided going to be bearable or unbearable for those who are fated to endure it? If some distinction could be made between bearable and unbearable suffering, a better case could be developed. The distinction, however, is patently difficult to make even with specific cases in view, and more difficult to make as a general one. The variables are many. One is relative to the consequences of the particular genetic disease under consideration. The consequences of having a Tay-Sachs infant are surely different from those caused by bearing a child with cleft palate or sickle cell anemia. The consequences of Huntington chorea are different from those of hypertension. By these observations we mean to suggest that some clue to a distinction between bearability and unbearability might be sought by attending to the consequences of the diseases, though in the end such a distinction will be relatively soft.

Another variable rests in the capacities of persons to tolerate suffering. Here both a person assessing his own capacities and an external observer assessing them are in the soft terrain of making estimates and predictions; absolutely firm judgments are almost impossible. There are significant differences between the forms of suffering, however, in this regard. If the financial assets and the earning power of a family with high risk for bearing children with a genetic disease whose therapy is costly are known, for example, some rather firm judgments can be made about the economic bearability of having an affected child. (Whether parents ought to be the exclusive bearers of such cost, or whether public resources ought to be made available to them to assist in bearing it, is a matter of the social ethics and social policy of medicine. To affirm the latter, which we would do, is also to open the door to a claim by public agencies to have a voice in the decisions of parents; that is, since the "public" is going to bear part of the cost, and since the "public" does not readily recognize a duty to bear costs that are avoidable, a public authority might claim a right to prohibit parents from bearing children who are great expense to the state or to philanthropic institutions.)

The capacity to bear physical pain is variable relative to the persons who are involved. When the persons involved are "persons" who *might* be born, the firmest ground for a discussion of bearability of pain is the evidence gained from persons who do suffer from the disease in question.

The capacity of persons to bear anxiety is the most difficult of all to judge. Individual differences are important and difficult to assess with precision. Also, the capacities of persons to bear anxieties and suffering alter through time and in different specific circumstances. Even when relatively objective evidence about the consequences of a genetic disease for the infant can be given, parents will respond to that information differently. A physician who has counseled parents might well have good clues about their capacities to bear the anguish involved in raising an affected child, but his perceptions might sometimes be inaccurate. Persons sometimes respond with unexpected fortitude, and sometimes with unexpected anger or despair. An element of prediction is always involved, since various contingencies and future experiences can alter the conditions in which families live and their capacities to bear the anguish of having a defective child. Some persons have come to bear suffering and anguish that they did not believe they could bear; some persons who have great capacities to bear anguish can dramatically lose those capacities as a result of unanticipated and untoward events in their lives. Judgments about the bearability of anxiety involved in raising an affected child are always uncertain.

Not only are such judgments difficult to make about parents and other family members; they are even more difficult to make about an infant who might be affected with a genetic disease. Again, specific issues would emerge with specific diseases or defects, and assessments of their severity are important to make. Since the conditions that make for more or less satisfactory emotional adjustment to a disability are multiple – the relations a child has with parents and sibs, his relations to peers in the community, the availability of care which can take into account the defect the child has, etc. – any prediction made will have to be within a rather wide range of probabilities.

Once the procedure has been established for justifying programs of genetic screening and the actions that might follow, on the basis of benefits, there is no way of avoiding the difficulties involved in judging potential consequences. Since the avoidance of suffering is a consequence that is sought, the difficulties of judging the severity of suffering, the bearability of suffering and other matters cannot be avoided. The problems involved in assessing bearability and unbearability of suffering must be faced in making judgments about benefits and costs. Alertness to the difficulties is important.

Another question that can be pressed on using the warrant of avoidance of suffering as a justification for genetic therapy is this: is a person morally free to avoid inconvenience and suffering for himself at the cost of causing suffering or even the elimination of life to others? A general answer to this question would find wide agreement. Persons are not under a moral obligation to undertake voluntarily most forms of suffering that they can avoid. For example, if a family is itself free from serious genetic defects, this does not (in any special sense) obligate it to adopt a Down syndrome child. This is not to claim that no one is under obligation to give the best possible care to such a child, nor even to claim that the parents of the child have sole responsibility for his care.

Answers to the question in more specific circumstances, however, become more complex. Are the parents of a diagnosed Tay-Sachs fetus morally free to avoid suffering for themselves and for their fetus at the cost of the life of the fetus? Most informed persons would agree that they are; the reasons given in support of such a judgment pertain specifically to the characteristics of the disease. If science and technology developed so that sickle cell anemia could be routinely diagnosed prenatally, the judgment *might* be different: the disease is not as severe; the life expectancy is greater; and while there is no cure for it, knowledge that the person has the disease can be used beneficially in his health care. It is also conceivable that many persons would make the same judgment that is generally made with reference to a Tay-Sachs fetus, but the grounds for the judgment would be different. They might be the following: the fetus does not have the rights and values of a person in any case; thus to abort a fetus is no serious sacrifice or cost. Since the particular fetus in question has a genetic disease, there is even more than the ordinary ground for eliminating its life.

In the past, at least, persons or families who have undertaken suffering voluntarily for the sake of others have generally been admired. Their action would be an instance of "self-sacrificial" morality, of going beyond the requirements of their rational self-interest to "walk the second mile." A distinction is not always easily made, however, between a self-sacrificial action and relationship on the one hand, and a clearer duty that a relationship might involve between a person who might be freed from suffering and one who would bear the cost of that freedom on the other hand. For example, the natural duty of parents to care to the best of their ability for their growing children cannot be violated without moral reproach. Parents who might feel that the anguish involved in raising adolescent children is costly cannot sever their relationships with their children for the sake of avoiding suffering. Their social role, the mutual dependencies involved in that role, and their causal responsibility in bringing children into the world carry with them duties (if not obligations) to suffer for the sake of their children. If this is recognized, it is fair to examine whether similar duties are present during pregnancy. If it is judged that they are not, some reasons must be given to account for the difference.

The crucial observation that would account for the difference is that age and time count in some way to make elimination of fetal life a different case. The importance of the age or time factor can be vividly noted by raising the following question. Is there a difference in the duties and obligations that parents have to bear the suffering involved in raising a child whose illness is detected after birth from their duties and obligations to bear and raise a child whose genetic disease is prenatally detected? The question is not a hypothetic one, since there are a significant number of instances in which neonates genetically defective – or at least congenitally affected with a polygenic disorder (eg myelomeningocele) – are permitted to die. An argument in favor of the moral significance of the distinction could be made only on the grounds that the age of the life involved counts, with its greater independence from the mother. Infanticide, including passive neglect of an infant, would be judged morally wrong, whereas abortion would be judged to be morally permissible. The cost involved in taking the infant's life for the sake of relieving its family from suffering (as defined in the particular set of circumstances) would be too great. But would it be too great to relieve the infant's future suffering? The infant, by virtue of having been born alive, would have to be judged to have a claim on parents that they have a duty or obligation to fulfill. The question would then have to be faced: if abortion of a prenatally detected diseased fetus is permissible, but not the infanticide of a defective neonate, why? Because the fetus has not been born? Because the neonate has certain degrees of independence that the fetus does not? Because there is a different relationship between parents and a neonate from that between parents and a fetus? The fact that distinctions are made in the stages of development from conception to maturity which do seem to count in making judgments about what actions are permissible to relieve the suffering of some persons at the cost of suffering and death to others, can be clearly established. However, the reasons that persons would give to justify the importance of the distinctions as data in judgments about procedures are seldom persuasive to all rational men.

Particular Anxieties That Might Be Raised by Genetic Screening

Whether the fact of being screened for genetic diseases raises anxieties that are burdensome is a matter that needs some discussion. There is no question that having medical information about oneself which signals actual or potential difficulties raises anxieties in most persons. But how persons cope with such information and anxiety is a matter of great individual variation. To know, for example, that one has a disease, genetic or nongenetic, for which there is no presently available therapy requires some personal and emotional coping. One might govern one's activity according to limitations which lessen the likelihood of crises, and thus perhaps prolong life; one might also be adversely affected by the uncertainty about one's future, and require not only medical but psychiatric care.

A particular instance in which anxieties might be intensified is that of persons who are detected to be carriers of a disease, and informed about the risks for their offspring, but have moral scruples about fulfilling the courses of action that might prevent affected children. A very orthodox Jewish family, for example, might believe that abortion is against the Jewish law; if the parents are carriers of Tay-Sachs disease their anxieties about bearing children would be intensified because the most feasible course of action to prevent the birth of an affected child is ruled out for them. Whether not to be informed about being a carrier through screening and possibly bearing an affected child would produce "less" anxiety is, of course, a matter that cannot accurately be assessed.

The fundamental issue is how well patients can manage information gained about themselves through screening. One variable in this is certainly the quality of the counseling that goes with screening. Even with effective counseling, however, diffuse anxieties about oneself and about one's progeny can be raised. Anxiety about progeny, however, is not a novel phenomenon; families with histories of hemophilia, for example, have lived with such concerns for a long time. The crucial practical question is whether the possibility of raising diffuse anxieties "outweighs" the potential benefits to those who become informed. Would a physician ever be justified, for example, in withholding information about being a carrier of hemophilia or Duchenne muscular dystrophy from a woman who is unaware of her risk and plans to have children? It is clear in these instances that the possible consequences of having affected children "outweighs" the possible benefits of freedom from anxiety based upon ignorance, that thus the answer to the question as specifically formulated here is negative.

Anxiety, we have noted, is a form of suffering, and thus to live is to be anxious. It is not clear that the anxieties that information about oneself and family gained through genetic screening might create are of sufficient magnitude to warrant restraint from being screened on those grounds alone. What is clear is that genetic screening without adequate genetic counseling to facilitate the comprehension of the information and its significance for the future is a mistake.

False Expectations

New medical information and technologies always tend to raise the expectations of patients, or even prospective patients, that they and their progeny can live free from diseases that men formerly endured. Screening might well raise the same sort of expectations. The avoidance of such false expectations, however, is a matter of the education and counseling that accompanies genetic screening; screening *per se* ought not to be judged wrong because of that possibility. To make clear to parents that the possibility of having a child who is free from one genetic disease does not imply that they will have a perfectly healthy child is part of the educational and counseling tasks that accompany genetic screening programs.

To assess any medical program in terms of its potential benefits or harm to persons (and every medical program exists for the sake of benefits) involves judgments about the consequences of procedures. Genetic screening is no exception. When the benefits to be assessed are not in the strictest sense simply biologic or medical benefits, but include wider aspects of the well-being of patients, families and society, a process is required that is complex, difficult and indeed slippery. We have indicated some aspects of the complexity and difficulty. To see the difficulties, however, is not to deny the importance of making concerted efforts to make the best possible assessments, with the best possible distinctions in mind. It might be intellectually neater, and rationally more persuasive, to devise a mode of making ethical judgments which could avoid the ambiguities involved in the assessment of benefits. It is likely, however, that such a procedure of analysis might mask some of the difficulties admitted in the one we have used simply by ruling them out of discussion as being "nonmoral." It has not been our purpose to engage in the refinements of what constitutes a moral value in distinction from a nonmoral value. Rather, it has been our purpose to alert the reader to some of the inherent issues involved in making judgments about genetic screening programs in terms of human values.

Acknowledgment

Valuable critical comments on an earlier draft were received during a meeting of the Hastings "Genetics Core Group," and particularly from written communications from Richard Erbe, M.D., Richard Roblin, Ph.D. and Marc Lappé, Ph.D.

References

1. Murdoch, I.: Vision and choice in morality. In Ramsey, I. (ed.): *Christian Ethics and Contemporary Philosophy.* New York:Macmillan Publishing Company, Inc., 1966, pp. 204ff.
2. Cunningham, G. C.: Phenylketonuria testing – Its role in pediatrics and public health, CRC Critical Reviews. *Clin. Lab. Sci., 2*:44-101, 1971.
3. Kaback, M. M. and Zeiger, R. S.: The John F. Kennedy Institute Tay-Sachs program: Practical and ethical issues in an adult genetic screening program. In Hilton, B., Callahan, D. et al (eds.): *Ethical Issues in Human Genetics.* New York:Plenum Press, 1973, pp. 131-146.

Ethical Issues in Genetic Screening

Models of Genetic Responsibility

Sumner B. Twiss, Jr., M.A., M.Phil., Ph.D.

Introduction

Despite the allure of remarkable developments in genetic engineering and the prospective problems they generate, certain current practices based on this technology pose urgent ethical and social issues which warrant immediate consideration.[1] One practical result of this knowledge and technology can be seen in the advent of many new types of genetic screening programs being established in order to help ensure the birth and development of healthy children. At least three types of screening programs are becoming increasingly prevalent in the practice of medical genetics: postnatal screening for the newborn, intrauterine amniocentesis for pregnant women and screening for carriers of deleterious genetic traits. The benefits of such genetic screening are easy to cite. For example, individuals or couples found to be at high risk for transmitting a serious genetic disease to potential offspring can take this information into account in making responsible decisions about procreation. In some instances, means are available for enabling them to bear unaffected children, by detecting through amniocentesis affected fetuses before birth and selectively aborting them. Thus the primary benefits of genetic screening can be conceived in terms of reducing the occasions for human suffering and tragedy, and in some cases providing opportunities for joy and happiness through the birth of healthy children. However, the benefits provided by genetic screening are only a part of the picture. The problems raised by such programs must also be considered.

Some very broad concerns include the following: Who has the legitimate authority to determine how the new genetic technology should be used? Scientists and physicians? Legislators? What are the proper ends for the use of this technology? For example, should this technology be

---

Sumner B. Twiss, M.A., M.Phil., Ph.D., *Assistant Professor, Department of Religious Studies, Brown University, Providence, R.I.*

employed in the service of parental desires to predetermine the sex of offspring? Will the pursuit of these ends on a societal level conflict with traditionally recognized human rights and values? If so, how does one weigh the rights of the individual against social needs and goods? For example, should eugenic considerations be allowed to override the human rights of self-determination in marrying and in founding a family? Does the potential of this technology imply new rights and values which ought to be recognized? For example, does every child have the right to begin life with a sound mind and body? These, among others, are quite legitimate and pressing issues.

Often it is fruitful to examine such broad concerns in association with a specific concrete development, such as the appearance of genetic screening programs. In fact, the issues raised by this development in medical genetics replicate on a smaller scale precisely the concerns just mentioned. It seems clear enough that inasmuch as it relates to the reproductive interests of prospective parents, genetic screening contains an element of man's attempt to guide his biologic future. In short, even this modest use of human genetics to reduce human suffering and improve the quality of human life by simply expressing active concern for the genetic quality of prospective children raises quite fundamental issues concerning legitimate authority, proper ends, conflicts between the individual and society, and so forth. For example, by what authority does the prospective parent have the right to decide who shall live or die, or what kind of person should be permitted to be born? Is it justifiable for parents or society to articulate standards of normalcy – to define "normal" – and to decide who shall be born on the basis of genetic make-up? Does society have a legitimate stake in trying to prevent genetic disease through the implementation of mandatory screening programs? Should legal constraints regarding procreation be imposed on individuals found to be at high risk for transmitting a serious genetic disease to potential progeny? It should be noted that attempting to answer such questions as these also involves trying to define notions basic not only to medicine but to human life in general: personhood, conditions of human welfare, normalcy, health, disease and what is properly construed as an acceptable quality of life – indeed an arduous task.

The principal focus, then, of the major ethical and social issues raised by genetic screening and correlated technologies is on qualitative decisions regarding human reproduction. There is an emerging concern on the part of the medical profession, parents, families and society for the biologic quality, or more specifically the genetic constitution, of future children.

The articulation of this concern is directly related to man's increased capacity to participate actively in determining certain aspects of the genetic quality of offspring. Although such intervention is still limited to the act of bearing or not bearing a child, genetic screening of carrier status and intrauterine diagnostic technics have injected new factors into reproductive decision-making and behavior. Now, on the basis of probability calculations, risk figures pertaining to the genetic constitution of potential children, decisions to avoid conceiving certain kinds of children can be made. Moreover, with access to intrauterine diagnosis and selective abortion, it is possible to select from unborn progeny and allow to come to term only those free from certain detectable genetic disorders. (See the paper by Kaback et al in this series.)

A significant theme which has surfaced precisely because of this increased capacity to intervene in determining the biologic quality of progeny is that of genetic responsibility. This theme is constantly touched on and variously articulated, but it has never been investigated systematically. References to the notion range from "squarely facing responsibility to the next generation" to "accepting responsibility for the germ plasm," culminating in "the right of every child to be born free from genetic defect and abnormality" or, alternatively, "the right of every child to begin life with a sound mind and healthy body."

These frequent but relatively undeveloped references to genetic responsibility suggest a particularly fruitful framework for elucidating a significant range of sociomoral issues raised by the practice of genetic screening. By developing a typology of major approaches to genetic responsibility, heuristic models can be adduced for exploring certain moral dimensions of this application of human genetics in which the demands of social institutions impinge on individual values and responsibility. Attention will be focused on the rights and duties of various social groups concerned with the genetic quality of their members, for example, the family, civil society, ethnic populations and the human species. The notion of a parental role, conceived as a common denominator in the concern of these groups, will be helpful in this investigation because it enables the ideas of institutional rights and duties to be combined and contrasted with those of individual responsibility and values. The hope is that this approach will expose significant tensions between individual values and institutional demands generated by medical genetics, or more specifically genetic screening. The predominant aim of this inquiry will be to provide an analytic and empiric account of emerging conceptions of genetic responsibility in order to explore their social and moral implications. A secondary goal is to lay some preliminary groundwork for proposing a minimal "ethic of genetic responsibility," that is, for making some normative remarks in the advocacy of a particular moral position.

The bulk of the following comments attempts to construct a framework for highlighting some major ethical and social issues in genetic screening. This endeavor is essentially descriptive rather than prescriptive in character. In particular, this inquiry is aimed at specifying certain conceptions of genetic responsibility that are emerging in our society. These views are approached from the perspective of the individual genetically screened. Considerable attention will be given to the moral aspects of the screenee's social roles as these bear on the development of concern for the genetic quality of progeny. To structure and facilitate this discussion, several working models of genetic responsibility will be elaborated. These models are offered as expository and heuristic devices for better understanding the emergent notions of genetic responsibility and for examining certain related ethical issues in genetic screening. The descriptive study of these emergent conceptions may also contribute to another sort of inquiry. More specifically, the models of genetic responsibility may help to further our understanding of the causal development of genetic screening programs and the societal or psycho-social pressures which these programs generate.

Although the main thrust of this investigation is descriptive and analytic in nature, since accepting its findings does not entail any normative commitment, the descriptive inquiry may be viewed as relevant to normative ethics. For example, a systematic study of these conceptions of genetic responsibility may suggest particularly appropriate ways of approaching and solving certain moral problems and thereby prompt the advocacy of one or another ethical perspective. In the concluding section some prescriptive comments will be sketched and briefly defended. These comments are made in the spirit of trying to crystallize what many might agree to as minimally acceptable components of genetic responsibility on the part of the individual screenee.

Categories of Analysis

Developing a helpful framework of analysis involves at least three main steps. First, the notion of responsibility must be explored within the horizons set by applied human genetics, in particular genetic screening. Second, in order to give some material content to this framework, certain implications of the principle of the sanctity of life need to be examined, again within the context of applied human genetics. Third, these explorations should provide materials sufficient enough to elucidate significant conceptions of genetic responsibility.

The notion of responsibility is most profitably analyzed in relation to the general concept of a sociomoral role, for responsibility is closely tied to the concepts of role, duty and obligation. Of course, the morality of role acceptance cannot be simply reduced to a description of the social role which is accepted by a person, for he is held responsible for the role which he accepts in the first place. Therefore, a person's responsibility cannot be completely and exhaustively analyzed in terms of the rights and duties constitutive of a social role. But it still remains true that responsibility is ordinarily attributed to an agent operating within a social role which prescribes certain duties. Roughly speaking, to be responsible is for such an agent to take his duties seriously, to see the point of fulfilling his duties, to adjust the performance of his duties to diverse circumstances and to act with discretion and fittingness in performing his duties. To the extent that such an agent is charged with the task of adjusting or fitting his duties to complex situations, he is held accountable not only for performing his duties but also for the propriety with which he interprets his duties in light of ambiguous, trying and novel circumstances. Furthermore, the mention of the agent's accountability indicates that the concept of responsibility is inherently transitive. That is, responsibility always involves accountability for (doing) something and accountability to someone (with a claim). Thus we speak of a person's being responsible for something in the sense that it is his task or role to deal with it, and we speak of a person's being responsible to another person or to a social group.[2]

It has often been noted that this transitive sense of role-responsibility presupposes another more basic sense of responsibility which involves an agent's free and rational ability to make his own decisions, to make up his own mind about what to do. This sense is obviously relevant to any adequate analysis of responsibility within the frame of a sociomoral role. This basic sense of responsibility refers to those capacities which must be possessed by an agent in order to speak of his being morally responsible for his actions. A person is morally responsible for his actions if he freely performs them with full knowledge of what he is doing. The conditions involved here include the capacities to understand what one is required to do, to be aware of relevant facts, to deliberate and decide what to do and to conform one's conduct to decisions made. These several capacities render a person morally responsible for his actions and enable us to speak of morally responsible as contrasted with morally irresponsible actions, and of liability for blame. These criteria for establishing attributions of moral responsibility can be more precisely formulated in terms of negative tests or excusing conditions, but the general sense ought to be clear enough.[3]

In the subsequent inquiry attention will be concentrated on the obligatory features (duties) of the notion of responsibility, although a full explication of responsibility requires a brief examination of the rights implied by a sociomoral role. In general, rights and duties are correlative notions. On the whole, rights derive from a context of regulative rules, for example, a sociomoral role, which specifies that a constitutive right implies a correlative duty on the part of other persons not to interfere with an agent's exercise of that right, or perhaps another person's duty to fulfill some obligation to the agent, as to keep a promise. Of course, this view of rights does not exhaust the nuances of our ordinary uses of "right;" however, two points are established. First, rights and duties are generally correlative notions. Second, the notion of right acquires its primary significance from normative contexts, such as sociomoral roles, which are themselves comprehended in terms of rules defining and regulating relationships among persons. One further point about rights which is relevant to the inquiry involves the notion of human rights, the basic rights which belong to persons as persons. These rights are characteristically universal and supreme. All persons have them by virtue of their common humanity, and they are considered to be of paramount importance to human life. Obvious examples of such human rights include life, liberty, equality and the pursuit of happiness.[4]

In the context of genetic screening, this brief analysis of responsibility raises such questions as the following with regard to the screenee: How is his sociomoral role to be defined? What duties or obligations are implied by this role? For what is he accountable? To whom is he accountable? When may he be said to act in a morally irresponsible fashion? These questions may not be exhaustive, but they are relevant and suggestive and provide valid points of orientation. Plausible answers to such questions are diverse, because the possible roles are many and overlapping. Examples include parent, family members, ethnic community member and species member. Depending upon which role or nexus of roles is emphasized, implied duties, rights and conceptions of responsibility may vary. In light of this diversity and variability, it may be most productive to select certain paradigmatic role conceptions or models for further investigation. Specifically, it may prove quite fruitful to explore five particular conceptions of the screenee's role and see what approaches to genetic responsibility are implied: parent simpliciter, parent-family member, parent-citizen, parent-ethnic population member and parent-species member.

The question may arise as to why the parental role is selected as a common denominator for these five paradigmatic models. There are a number of reasons for emphasizing the parental role and focusing attention on the reproductive aspects of applied human genetics. First, whether rightly or wrongly, it appears that the success of genetic screening and counseling programs has been and will continue to be assessed, at least in part, in terms of their impact on the reproductive decisions and behavior of parents and prospective parents. Second, the objective or rationale for genetic screening cited by many programs is precisely to enhance the quality of parental choices in reproduction: the provision of genetic information widens parental options, enriches the decision-making process and enlarges parents' freedom of choice and self-determination. Third, on the face of it, it seems that the basic thrust of such programs is to encourage genetic intervention on the part of parents and prospective parents in their reproductive behavior so as to prevent the birth of children with serious genetic defects. Finally, inasmuch as the locus of man's active participation in shaping his biologic future inevitably crosses paths with the highly valued role of parenthood, it makes good sense to focus on parenthood and reproduction even when looking beyond the nuclear family and, for example, taking stock of societal considerations.

In attempting to elucidate the conceptions of genetic responsibility implied by the five selected role models, it may be helpful to examine certain aspects of the principle of the sanctity of life. There are several reasons for selecting and examining this principle in the context of the present inquiry. One reason involves an empiric observation about its consensual character and historical role in our pluralistic society. On the basis of this principle, fundamental moral rules and human rights regarding human welfare and happiness have been formulated, recognized and justified. A second reason is related to the first but makes a stronger claim. Given certain premises, indeed truisms, about the nature of man and his environment, any stable society must institutionalize certain types of moral rules and rights based on this principle, basic rules of social life which promote conditions of human welfare. A third reason involves a more ambitious philosophic claim. It argues that the very existence of practical reasoning and the logic of practical discourse pertaining to the basic problems of human conduct presuppose certain fundamental principles which form a distinctive and coherent moral point of view; one of these principles is the sanctity of life. A fourth and quite pragmatic reason is that many people in our culture accept this principle as a valid point of departure for discussing sociomoral issues. A consensus on its usefulness and validity already exists, so why not capitalize on this widespread recognition? As a point of departure, the principle may be formulated in alternative ways, for example, as an injuntion to render due respect to human life, as an injunction to affirm and respect all human life or as an injunction to treat all human life as if it were sacred.[5]

The principle has both a material value in implying certain general directives for conduct and a legitimating function as a procedural principle of interpretation in moral deliberation and justification. That is, the principle has two aspects, one prescriptive and the other procedural. It provides general prescriptions about conduct by delimiting a range within which an agent may exercise his discretion with regard to human life. For example, the principle clearly establishes a presumption against the taking of human life. Moreover, the manner in which the principle is primarily used indicates that its function and utility is procedural in character. It is meant to be employed as a high-level justificatory principle in situations of deliberation about rules and rights relating to intervention in the human life process. In other words, the principle is a basic validating norm which establishes general limits of action regarding human life. While the content of the principle is open-ended in the sense that it is subject to discretionary interpretation and application in concrete situations, it specifies clear reference points for its proper application. It is understood always to rule against certain kinds of action, like the arbitrary taking of human life, and always to encourage other sorts of action, like promoting the survival and protection of human life. These outer negative and positive limits still leave much to the discretion of individuals and social groups faced with specific decisions, but the point is that general limits of action are indicated, or more strongly implied. On the whole, the principle establishes a firm presumption that human life ought to be protected against destructive intervention. Since intervention in the process of human life may occur at a number of points, for example, relating to the individual person, the family and the human species; at least three significant clusters of moral rules, rights and values are implied by the principle. These clusters pertain to the integrity and material welfare of the person, the family and the human species. They may be introduced briefly as follows.

The integrity of the person is specified by two general principles or rules which may be tagged "nonmaleficence" and "consideration."

Nonmaleficence proscribes killing or inflicting pain on other persons. Phrased positively, it enjoins that every person be allowed to live and enjoy the protection of others. Consideration proscribes arbitrary interference by others in the self-determined destiny of an individual. More positively, it enjoins persons to make allowances in their own plans for the self-determined life concerns of others. The sense of both rules is encapsulated in the notion of the human right to life, that is, a right to life with a distinctively human quality. It is stipulated here that qualitatively human life is distinctively personal life which is had in virtue of an individual's ability to exercise self-determination or free agency. The integrity of the family involves an extension of the rules of nonmaleficence and consideration to proscriptions on the arbitrary termination of family lineages and on arbitrary interference in the founding, planning and preservation of families. Phrased positively, individuals and families should be allowed to propagate children, plan the size of families and perpetuate family lineages. The sense of these rules is captured in the notion of a human right to marry and found a family. Obviously included in this right are the rights of self-determination in procreation, becoming a parent and continuing family lineage. The integrity of the human species further extends the rules of nonmaleficence and consideration so that individuals and social groups are prohibited from endangering the life of the species, both present and future. Phrased positively, individuals and social groups are enjoined to act so as to maintain the existence of the species and to provide a viable life for future generations. Unlike the other clusters of moral rules regarding the individual and the family, there is no clear-cut corresponding human right since there is no clear locus for a claim of noninterference. A case can be argued, however, that future generations have a claim against present generations, thus suggesting a human right of species preservation.

This brief discussion of the principle of the sanctity of life and the derived clusters of moral rules and rights will help structure the examination of the five roles selected for inquiry. It should be obvious that the integrity of the person, the family and the species has some bearing on genetic interventions contemplated by or on behalf of parents, families, civil society, ethnic populations and the species.

Five Models of Genetic Responsibility

Drawing upon these introductory discussions of responsibility and the principle of the sanctity of life, it is now possible to articulate five significant conceptions of genetic responsibility from the perspective of the genetic screenee. Since all five models have the parental role as a common denominator, it serves as an appropriate point of departure.

Parental Role

The first model of genetic responsibility involves examining parental role-responsibility in the context of applied human genetics, or more precisely genetic screening. Defining the parental role is no simple matter. It seems clear that the role is grounded in very basic human rights related to the integrity of the person and the integrity of the family: the right to human life with a self-determined destiny, the right to marry and found a family, the right to voluntary procreation. The moral vantage point for understanding the basis of this sociomoral role simply involves recognizing the integrity and inviolability of each individual person insofar as these imply that a person has the right to make decisions about his life development in interpersonal relations, which of course include sexual relations. Reproductive decisions, which form the heart of the parental role, are therefore expressions of prospective parents' rights to exercise control over events which are of major importance in their personal life development. Such decisions and rights do not exhaust the sociomoral dimensions of parenthood. Something must be said about the notion of responsibility within the frame of this role. For example, parents are accountable for the welfare of their children, and in this regard they are accountable to their children and to certain civil authorities representing the children's interests.

Parental responsibility may be elucidated in part by the following minimal duty: to care for, support, sustain and otherwise contribute to the growth and development of the child, providing for his basic needs and welfare and preparing him to become a socialized individual. Alternative formulations of this basic duty may be adduced, but the main thrust is clear enough. (Implied constitutive duties to provide affection, protection, nourishment, clothing, shelter, education, etc. seem evident.[6])

The particularly interesting question is whether the parental role, ordinarily founded on certain biologic facts, implies any genetic duties. This question may be interpreted in a number of ways. Some formulations are much more plausible than others. For example, are prospective parents obligated by their sociomoral role to ensure, so far as possible, normal genotypes for their children? Since it is hard to know what counts as a "normal genotype" and it is biologically unrealistic to ask anyone to "ensure" that a child be born with one, a more plausible way of stating the issue is this: does parental role-responsibility imply the duty to avoid bearing children with serious genetic defects? This same issue may be stated in the language of rights: does every child have the right to be born free of serious genetic defect insofar as this can be achieved? The controversial points raised by these two questions include such problems as the following:

1. What counts as a "serious genetic defect"?
2. Is abortion for genetic indications justifiable?
3. If there is such a parental duty or child's right, then does not this imply that a parental decision to have a genetically affected child is morally irresponsible and blameworthy?
4. If so, then does not this duty or right come into direct conflict with parental rights of self-determination? How is this conflict to be resolved?

Granting the difficulties in answering these questions, it seems that an affirmative answer to the question of genetic duty might be plausibly argued. For example, it might be argued that consensus can be reached on which genetic diseases are clearly severe enough to be avoided. If so, then selective abortion for these genetic conditions might well be viewed as justifiable. A case might well be argued that with foreknowledge of the high risk and in face of the available option of selective abortion, a parental decision to conceive and then to knowingly bear a child with a serious genetic defect constitutes a morally irresponsible act. In spite of the controversial issues, it might well be argued that parental role-responsibility does imply certain basic genetic duties, such as avoiding wherever feasible the procreation of children with detectable serious genetic defects. Such a conception of genetic responsibility would imply the duty to be genetically screened under certain circumstances, for example, if one had reason to believe that he might be a carrier of a detectable deleterious genetic trait.

There is much evidence to support the contention that this notion of genetic responsibility is currently emerging and taking definite form. Naturally enough, parents do not desire to have defective or abnormal children. Many concerned parents are carefully planning for children; and because of perceived social expectation and pressure to produce a limited number of children, there is an increasing parental concern for the genetic health of each child. Moreover, because having a child increasingly can be an active and informed choice, parents will want to be sure that each child starts life as healthy and normal as possible. Thus, they are willing and even view it as obligatory to undergo genetic screening in order to better the odds for having a healthy and normal child. Parents undergoing intrauterine diagnosis and selective abortion are themselves invoking such rights as the right of the child to reasonable mental and physical health, the right to a good mental life, the right to be free of genetic defect, in justifying their decisions. (See the paper by Kaback et al in this series for statements representative of professionals.) So this first model of genetic responsibility is already extant and operative.[7]

Parent-Family Member Role

The second model of genetic responsibility involves examining parent-family member role-responsibility in the context of applied human genetics. This model pertains to the nexus of two roles and involves rights relating to the integrity of the family. A number of preliminary points need to be noted about both the social institution of the family and its normative dimensions. Briefly, a family may be conceived as an association of persons tied together by customary rules of kinship. It is, then, a kinship association whose members openly acknowledge and cooperate in the pursuit of mutual concerns, needs, desires and hopes. On this view it clearly makes sense to speak of duties, rights and responsibility within the family institution. But this is a somewhat attenuated notion of a family. In describing a family it is necessary not only to account for sociomoral relations but also to recognize the emotional bonds of preferential love, affection and loyalty which ground these moral relations.

It is true that kinship determines family membership, but the criteria of kinship and their importance are somewhat vague. How far does a family extend beyond the immediate circle of parents and children, the nuclear family? To grandparents, uncles and aunts? That seems reasonable enough. But how about second cousins and even more distant relatives? From the standpoint of human genetics, these are not idle questions by any means. An important observation to make about the family in our society is precisely its indeterminacy. Family "self" images, so to speak, are stipulated by the members themselves. That is, the significant boundaries of a family are family-specific. Moreover, in our society interest in genealogy, keeping up with extended family lineages, is on the decline. And note well that the range and extent of the sense of familial responsibility varies directly with the "self" definition of a particular family. It should be recognized that defining the family is itself an important sociomoral issue warranting some hard thinking. Human genetics points up the importance of this issue, for in many cases it is quite conceivable that the nuclear family may acquire genetic information relevant to the "genetic health" of more distant relatives and at the same time define family membership in such a way that duties to communicate with those relatives are simply not perceived.

This point raises the broader matter of how the rights and duties of family members are determined, how the familial role is to be specified. As in the case of the parental role simpliciter, it seems clear that the familial role is grounded in those basic human rights related to the integrity of the family. Recall that the central familial rules prescribe that families should be allowed to propagate children, plan family size and perpetuate their lineages as they choose and that these rules are encapsulated in corresponding human rights regarding procreation, parentage, founding and continuing a family. The moral vantage point for understanding the basis of this sociomoral role, therefore, simply involves recognizing the implications of the notions of family integrity and self-determination. Moreover, it would seem to be the case that the determination of any matter as a familial duty depends upon how important that concern is for the preservation of the life and welfare of the family. This point seems to follow from the notion of the integrity of the family and illuminates, at least in part, the character of responsibility within the frame of this role.

Consequently, the role-responsibility of a family member may be defined by the following minimal duty: to preserve the life of the family, contribute to its welfare and continue its lineage. A family member is accountable for this duty and its constitutive obligations, and he is accountable to other members of the family for their fulfillment. It is relatively easy to see that insofar as this familial role-responsibility involves or overlaps with the parental role, it may be argued that it includes certain basic genetic duties. One such duty is avoiding wherever feasible the procreation of children with detectable serious genetic defects who would exert a deleterious effect on the life and welfare of the family by draining its resources and terminating potential lines of lineage. Such a conception of genetic responsibility would also imply the duty to be genetically screened under certain conditions, again for example, if one had reason to believe that he might be a carrier of a detectable deleterious genetic trait.

It may also be argued that the familial role implies certain genetic duties beyond those possibly included in parental role-responsibility. On the ground of preserving the life and welfare of the family, it may be argued that every family member has the general obligation to inform other relevant family members of matters relating to their welfare and more broadly to the value of preserving the family. Inasmuch as genetic concerns may impinge on such welfare and value, it can be argued that family members have the genetic duties to ascertain whether they are carriers of a recessive genetic condition with serious medical consequences, at least if they suspect that they might be carriers of a seriously defective genetic trait, and to inform relevant family members about certain features of their genetic make-up, particularly if this information is relevant to the welfare of other members or the family as a whole. Again, this aspect of familial genetic responsibility would seem to imply the duty to be genetically screened in certain circumstances, not only to avoid procreating seriously defective children but also to help other family members to avoid such procreation.

There is evidence to support the contention that this notion of genetic responsibility also is emerging and taking definite shape. The experience of genetic counselors clearly indicates that parents assess genetic information – risk figures, severity of the disease, factors of chronic pain, mental retardation, morbidity, etc. – from the perspective of its potential total impact on the family. In figuring medical costs, frequency of hospitalization, the prospect of institutionalization, parents take into account such factors as prolonged distress for the family, effects on the welfare of extant children and effects on the financial resources of the nuclear and extended family. This sort of assessment clearly involves the recognition of genetically oriented familial responsibilities. Moreover, upon receiving genetic information many parents and prospective parents evidence a concern for relatives that may be possibly at high risk for carrying a recessive trait, and by implication recognize a duty to warn such relatives if this seems genetically indicated. There are, of course, problems concerning invasion of privacy, logistic problems in locating distant relatives and many situations in which screenees do not want to contact other family members. But these problems should not obscure the basic point that the duty to communicate genetic information, along with the broader conception of familial genetic responsibility, is indeed operative and viable.[8]

Parent-Citizen Role

The next three models of genetic responsibility involve examining parent-species member role-responsibility in the context of applied human genetics. At the outset it should be noted that there are three significant ways of developing a model along these lines. One approach examines the stake of civil society in human genetics. A second approach works on the notion of differentiated populations within the society and within the human species as a whole. A third approach works on an undifferentiated conception of the human species. Since each of these approaches suggests distinctive, albeit related, models of genetic responsibility, they will be developed independently. The basis for all three models is grounded in the notion of the integrity of the human species which prohibits individuals and social groups from endangering the life of the species, enjoins them to maintain the existence of the species and to provide a viable life for future generations, and suggests that there may be a human right of species preservation. Insofar as these rules and the corresponding right may be conceived as applicable respectively to civil societies, ethnic populations, and the human species as a whole, it may be suggested that the moral vantage point for understanding the roles of parent-citizen, parent-ethnic population member and parent-species member within the context of human genetics is sufficiently similar in all three cases that subsequent attention may be focused on the nuanced conceptions of genetic responsibility implied by each.

Thus, the third model of genetic responsibility involves examining parent-citizen role-responsibility in the context of applied human genetics. At first glance it might seem that the construction of this model is somewhat farfetched, but pause for a moment and reflect on the state's traditional interest in the family. Note that the state has built up an elaborate legal structure relating to the family, prescribing minimum ages for marriage, prohibiting marriage between close relatives and regulating certain aspects of child rearing. These observations suggest that the parental role, the nuclear function of the family, is of interest to others besides parents and relatives alone. Citizens in general have an interest in the exercise of the parental role, for it is a matter of public concern that progeny be equipped to become useful members of society.

The common life of the family proceeds within the larger community of the state. As members of that larger community, namely as citizens, parents naturally identify with what may be called the "ideal image" of the state association. Through that image they develop a loyalty to the larger community and its members, their fellow nationals. This bond of loyalty provides, at least in part, the foundation for the role of citizen. Without engaging in complex issues of political philosophy, it may be said that the role-responsibility of the citizen is elucidated by the following minimal duty: to help further the common good and to act in the public interest. The citizen is accountable for those of his actions which affect the public welfare, and he is accountable to other citizens and to the state's legal authorities.

The issue of a citizen's genetic responsibility as both parent and citizen represents relatively unexplored terrain. But there are signs that indicate the significance and seriousness of this issue. To begin with, it should be noted that civil society appears to take a substantial interest in both the quantity and quality of children born within the larger community. This interest is clearly evidenced by the development of publicly supported family planning programs, provision of contraceptive services, national commissions on population control and the like on the one hand, and legal requirements concerning mandatory education, court decisions ordering medical care for children against parental wishes, laws and court decisions in the area of child abuse, etc. on the other hand (See the paper by Green and Capron in this series.) In these and other ways, the state is expressing societal interest in the quantity and quality of the progeny of its citizenry. It is not wholly implausible to suggest that this interest is integrally tied up with the social utilitarian aims of maximizing the number of socially useful people and minimizing the number of socially burdensome people. In terms of health, these aims materialize in a public interest in ensuring that future citizens are healthy and a public interest in avoiding the costs involved in caring for defective, incapacitated persons.

There are clear signs that society is directly concerned with the genetic quality of prospective citizens. For example, a small number of genetic diseases are thought to be common enough to generate a public health concern. (Cf Green and Capron in this series.) Whether rightly or wrongly, then, genetic disease is sometimes conceived as a public health issue. Moreover, there is some indication that participation in certain genetic screening programs will be made legally mandatory by the enactment of public statutes. (See the paper by Powledge in this series.) The growing recognition that the consequences of some serious genetic diseases affect what is commonly called the public interest is distinct from but somewhat related to the public health issue. For example, public funds are used in researching therapies and providing institutional care.

These signs and the judgment of public health concern have been rejected as unjustifiable, on the grounds that genetic diseases are neither contagious nor, for the most part, susceptible to treatment at present. But that sort of counterargument overlooks three important points. First, many population geneticists do in fact agree that some genetic diseases are matters of public health hazard. Second, genetic diseases do affect the public interest through the social allocation of public funds and medical resources. Third, the argument fails to recognize its own contingent character and thereby also fails to address the issue of principle regarding a citizen's genetic responsibility. Thus it is valid to question whether the citizen's basic obligation to further the common good implies a subsidiary genetic duty, in light of the fact that genetic disease does affect the public interest and may possibly be a legitimate public health problem.

An affirmative response to this question is not wholly implausible. It may be argued that the parent-citizen's role-responsibility implies certain genetic duties, such as avoiding the procreation of children with serious genetic defects who might adversely affect the public welfare, for example, by using up much needed funds and scarce medical resources, and even the public health in light of their long-term effect on the gene pool. Such a conception of genetic responsibility would imply the duty to be genetically screened, under certain circumstances, in order to avoid the birth of genetically defective children.

Once again there is some evidence that such a conception of genetic responsibility is emerging within our society. Here, of course, one immediately thinks of certain views promulgated by population geneticists regarding the so-called pollution of the gene pool. While such views are relevant, the views of the public at large and the views of genetic screenees and counselees are much more germane. It is becoming ever more apparent from reading the popular press that there is an emerging public concern over the genetic quality of prospective citizens. Genetic disease is regarded as the biologic aspect of the escalating pollution problem. This perspective in turn has evoked public concern about the genetic quality of future generations of citizens which is expressed in terms of acting responsibly for what is in the wider public interest. The resulting social pressure for legislative action in the area of applied human genetics (genetic screening) is well known. The upshot of these developments is an emerging conception of a citizen's genetic responsibility along the lines reified in the above model. Moreover, this conception is sometimes exhibited in genetic counseling situations where parents themselves, not so much the counselors, raise questions about the eugenic and social implications of their reproductive behavior. Such parental recognition of genetic obligations owed to the larger community is aptly symbolized by the felt duty to procreate so-called perfect children.[9]

Parent-Species Member Role

In order to get a sense of a fourth distinctive model of genetic responsibility, recall the notion of the integrity of the species – that the species ought to maintain itself in existence and as distinctively human, that the species ought to work toward its survival and, more pertinent, that present humans ought to act in such a way that they ensure, or at least do not endanger, a viable life for future members of the species. It may be argued that derivative from these rules regarding the integrity of the species is a conception of genetic responsibility on the part of present generations to future generations, which may be encapsulated in the genetic duty to avoid doing any act harmful to the basic genetic constitution of the human species. There are many problems inherent in this model. Determining what sort of genetic acts really harm the species and specifying the genetic harm are the biggest problems. Ascertaining what "accountability" can mean in this context is no minor difficulty either. Nevertheless, the fact that acts performed by one generation can significantly affect subsequent generations lends some credence to this model. If the procreation of children with serious genetic defects can be construed as a class of acts harmful to the species' genetic constitution, then the avoidance of such procreation can be argued as a genetic duty incumbent upon a parent-species member. This conception of genetic responsibility would also imply the duty to be genetically screened, under certain circumstances, in order to avoid the birth of genetically defective children.

There is some evidence that this conception of genetic responsibility, as distinct from the societal model, is taking shape. Again, one thinks of population geneticists and their view that the principal sociomoral issue in human genetics is that present generations should accept responsibility for the quality of the human gene pool or germ plasm over which they have temporary stewardship and will transmit to future generations. It must be recognized that this population perspective cuts across the boundaries of civil societies and national groups to the extent that people in many societies share a growing concern over mankind's movement in a so-called genetically apocalyptic age. It is not widely implausible to suggest that this widespread concern for the biologic quality of future generations is giving rise to a distinctive notion of genetic responsibility which many parents and prospective parents recognize and accept even from their individualistic outlook.[10]

Parent-Ethnic Population Member Role

The fifth model of genetic responsibility involves articulating a differential approach to the parent-species model. More precisely, it requires examining parent-ethnic population member role-responsibility in the context of applied human genetics. Certain facts bolster the potential significance of this model. The frequency of occurrence of certain genetic diseases can be correlated with identifiable "high-risk" populations. Moreover, some of these populations have a degree of community identity which might conceivably ground the mutual recognition of population-specific concerns and obligations. These facts suggest that certain aspects of the parent-family member, the parent-citizen and the parent-species member models of genetic responsibility may be combined to yield yet another distinctive model. The basic task would involve developing a conception of a definable population along species, social and familial lines. That is, a certain identifiable high-risk population could be regarded as a part of the species, as a social interest group and as a large "family." Duties for a population member implied by this conception would parallel those for the species member, the citizen and the family member as parent. For example, present population members ought to work for the population's welfare and maintain its distinctive heritage. Or more to the point, present population members ought to act so that they ensure a viable life for future population members, and members should act to preserve the life of the population and continue its heritage. In this view it would appear that a population member is accountable for those of his actions which affect the welfare, life and continuation of the population, and he is accountable to other population members.

In turn it may be argued that those duties which specify the role-responsibility of a population member imply certain basic genetic duties. Such duties may include avoiding the procreation of children with those serious genetic defects which are specific to the population, insofar as such procreation could be considered as harmful to both the present *and* future welfare of the population; ascertaining the make-up of one's genotype (ie finding out whether one is a carrier of a population-specific deleterious gene); and possibly imparting this genetic information to other population members under certain conditions, for example, before marriage. Certainly, such a conception of genetic responsibility would imply the duty to be genetically screened, under certain conditions, in order both to avoid procreating seriously defective children and to cooperate with other population members in helping them avoid the birth of seriously defective children.

The evidence for this distinctive conception of genetic responsibility is massive. One need only consider the positive response of black communities in our society to the development of genetic screening programs for the sickle cell trait. (See the paper by Powledge in this series.) Despite the problems of poor legislation in this matter, problems of social stigmatization and resulting discrimination, and even charges of genocide, it is undeniable that there is an increasing consciousness on the part of black communities that sickle cell anemia is a distinctively ethnic health problem which calls for responsible action – hence the black population's general support for development of sickle cell screening programs and even for legislative action in this area. Screening for carrier status is often regarded as a duty, and it is conceivable that many blacks believe that genetic information regarding carrier status for the sickle cell trait should be communicated not only to family members but also to prospective spouses before marriage. In other words, many blacks may believe that genetic information should be taken into consideration in mate selection.

Social Causes and Pressures

So far, five approaches to the theme of genetic responsibility have been distinguished and briefly developed, according to the roles of parent simpliciter, parent-family member, parent-citizen, parent-species member and parent-ethnic population member. Although these five models have not been fully developed, their preliminary articulation may help to provide some insight into the social causes for the development of genetic screening programs and to project what sort of social pressures may be generated by these programs.

The problem of identifying those social causes responsible for the development of genetic screening programs calls for extensive historical and sociologic investigation which cannot be undertaken here. However, perhaps some provisional suggestions may be made structured along the lines of these models of genetic responsibility. To begin with, the so-called logic of technologic expansion seems to be a relevant factor. Fallacious as it may seem, that "logic" involves two "principles" which appear to underlie technologic advances in our culture: because we can do something, we ought to gather together our resources and do it; and again, because we can do something, we inevitably will do it, so why wait on the development and implementation of rational social policy? It follows from this approach to technical development that feasibility may well have been one of the principal causes for the emergence of genetic screening programs.

The five models of genetic responsibility may help to identify other social factors which have increased and which will continue to increase the practical application of human genetics. First, the rapid advances in genetics and related biomedical technology have produced an almost euphoric ethos in our culture and society regarding the control and elimination of genetic diseases in the population (species model). These advances are suffusing our culture and society with an awareness of the genetic roots of certain diseases and have at least created an atmosphere of expectation that the medical control of these diseases is now possible or imminent. New scientific capabilities relating to family planning, population control and, more particularly, negative and positive eugenics have projected a conception of genetic responsibility to future generations into cultural and social consciousness. Such a sense of responsibility, no matter how amorphous, would be likely to back the development of genetic screening programs. In short, changes in cultural and societal attitudes and practices may be leading to a virtual demand for programs in applied human genetics. Second, genetic research into disease frequency in identifiable high-risk ethnic populations, together with related advances in carrier detection and therapies, has made genetic screening both feasible and desirable for certain ethnic communities (ethnic population model). Insofar as certain of these high-risk populations have some degree of community identity and organization, they are likely to develop a distinctive sense of genetic responsibility and to support genetic screening programs relevant to their respective medical problems. Third, the investment of public funds in medical-genetic research aimed at producing practical results has evoked the issue of public interest in genetic screening (citizen model). Inasmuch as the consequences of certain genetic diseases affect the public welfare in utilizing public funds for medical research and health care, the conception of the citizen's genetic responsibility begins to develop and become effective, for example, in the enactment of legal statutes regarding genetic screening. Finally, the growing use of genetic counseling clinics indicates that parents and prospective parents are beginning to assume some sort of genetic responsibility in regard to procreation and family welfare (parent and family models). Presumably, this assumption of responsibility affects, directly or indirectly, the development and growth of genetic screening programs. A related value consideration which may well contribute to the practical results in question involves the premium which parents in our society place on having "perfect" children. Such a valuation may well lead to the false, but still action-guiding expectation that supporting the new developments in applied human genetics will aid in producing the so-called dream child.

What social pressures are generated by genetic screening programs? Three of the five models of genetic responsibility appear particularly relevant to this question: the parent-citizen model, the parent-species member model and the parent-ethnic population member model. Once again, the answer to this question obviously requires sociologic research and prediction, but in lieu of protracted studies, common sense must suffice. What pressures, then, may be reasonably expected to develop? Expectations in light of the citizen model include increasing pressure toward viewing genetic screening as a public health concern, along with the possible emergence of governmental intervention in reproductive behavior. Expectations in light of the ethnic population model include the development of strong community psychosocial sanctions encouraging participation in those genetic screening programs relevant to corresponding high-risk populations, particularly those with a high degree of social or group identity. Expectations in light of the species model include the possible development of worldwide genetic screening programs sponsored by international health organizations. Predicting the social pressures related to genetic screening within the frame of these three models does not exhaust the question, however, for surely the parent and family models of genetic responsibility will generate distinctive pressures of their own, especially of a psychologic character. For example, the following sorts of developments may be anticipated: family encouragement of genetic screening and of imparting genetic information to relatives, or possibly the development of guilt feelings for not fulfilling parental and familial genetic duties.

The issue of social pressure needs to be explored even more thoroughly in regard to all five models of genetic responsibility. Such questions as the following merit consideration: Will genetic screening become a moral imperative? Will the practice of genetic screening develop in such a way that individuals will be screened against their wishes? Will families in which children with serious genetic defects are born feel guilty for having had such children? Will family members who are carriers of seriously defective genetic traits be made to feel responsible for informing relatives who might also be carrying those traits? The previous discussion obviously has some bearing on these questions. Within the frame of all five models, an affirmative answer to the question of moral imperativeness is not implausible. In the frames of the citizen, ethnic population and species models, an affirmative answer to the question of social coercion seems quite possible. Again, within the frame of all five models, an affirmative answer to the question of guilt feelings is certainly not implausible, especially with reference to genetic diseases which can be screened for in the carrier state and which have had widespread and well-publicized screening programs for a reasonable length of time. In the frame of the family model particularly, an affirmative answer to the question of feeling responsible for informing relatives seems quite plausible.

Ethical and Social Issues

A difficult question is whether these expected social pressures are justified or unjustified. That is, should they be encouraged or combatted? Posing this question raises the issue of appraising the models of genetic responsibility, inasmuch as these conceptions effect, at least in part, the predicted consequences regarding societal pressures. Such an assessment may be made on a number of grounds, for example, judging the internal clarity and consistency of each model, weighing the values, duties, obligations incorporated in each model against other conflicting human rights and values, and comparing the general cogency of each model to that of the other models. Although it is no easy task, a tentative and preliminary examination in light of these considerations may prove useful. This assessment will be divided into two parts. First, each model will be examined on its own merits, certain problems will be sighted and a provisional evaluation will be made. This initial assessment will also serve to develop the models more fully. The second section of the appraisal will be organized quite differently. Four central questions raised by three of the models in particular will be formulated, and then relevant considerations relating to these questions will be adduced, in order to provide a more detailed and mature assessment.

General Assessment of the Models

The parental model of genetic responsibility appears reasonably coherent. However, it does raise at least two internally controversial issues, one relatively minor and the other quite substantial. The minor problem concerns the claim that parents are accountable to their children for their children's welfare and for their potential children's welfare. Does this claim make sense? Although the issues cannot be finally settled here, the claim seems plausible with regard to extant children, especially in view of the fact that children are accorded moral, if not also legal, rights against their parents. It also makes some sense to discuss duties owed to potential children, insofar as prospective parents have some preconception of their children who have not yet been born. It is not wildly irresponsible, then, to accord children-to-be the moral and legal status of persons to whom parents can be held accountable, and it is not inconceivable to talk and reason about the welfare, rights and duties owed to potential children. The major issue internal to the parental model, and inherent in the other models also, involves defining those concepts basic to parental responsibility in a genetic context: health, disease, normalcy, personhood, welfare and the like. The fundamental question raised for this and the other models is whether it is justifiable to articulate standards of normalcy – to decide who shall be born – on the basis of genetic constitution. How does one go about arguing the case? This question will be addressed in the second part of the appraisal; at this point it may merely be noted that this is a difficult but not necessarily irresolvable issue. Does the parental model of genetic responsibility lead to conflicts with other important human rights or values? Taking into account the presumed right of voluntary procreation and all of its implications, the answer seems affirmative.

Thus, there is a *prima facie* conflict between the recommended parental genetic duty and the traditionally recognized right to voluntary procreation. However, this conflict is not irresolvable from the moral point of view. For example, it may be argued that the right to procreation is not an absolute right – most rights are not absolute – but rather one which is, or can be, circumscribed under certain conditions. Considering the increasingly widespread acceptance of population control, such an argument must have some plausibility: morally relevant circumstances for limiting the right of procreation are recognized. It is not inconceivable that these might be legitimately extended to include genetic considerations.

The parent-family member model of genetic responsibility is also reasonably coherent. Certain problems intrinsic to the familial model have already been indicated, particularly the very significant issue of how to determine the boundaries of a family. Are there any other problems internal to this model? Insofar as this model, like the others, proscribes the birth of children with serious genetic defects, it too raises the problem of defining basic concepts and justifying standards of normalcy. There are at least three further problems with this model, two internal and the other involving a conflict with traditional rights. One internal problem concerns the legitimacy of the value of preserving or continuing the family lineage. Is this value, along with its corresponding right, self-evidently implied or justified by the principle of the sanctity of life? The problem of trying to define the family would suggest otherwise. It appears that this value is being increasingly ignored, or not counted as a "value," in our society. Although empiric observations are certainly not decisive for moral matters, they are useful in singling out debatable points at the very least.

The other internal problem concerns the propriety of justifying, at least in part, the prohibition against bearing children with serious genetic defects on the basis of avoiding extraordinary costs to the family. From a moral perspective can economic considerations be viewed as having significant moral import? Can the avoidance of heavy expenditures of family resources be invoked with any decisiveness in moral deliberation over the weighty issues of human life? Answering such questions affirmatively would seem to suggest that the value of human life could be subjected to cost-benefit analysis. But should the value of human life, together with the right to life, ever be balanced against economic factors? At least in the present context, perhaps, this sort of reasoning can be viewed as morally licit, insofar as parental-familial responsibility involves consideration of the welfare of other family members, for example, taking account of duties owed to extant children. In this instance economic considerations could be construed as morally relevant factors inasmuch as they impinge on the welfare of other family members and may prevent the fulfillment of present obligations.

The third problem raised by the parent-family member model involves the *prima facie* conflict between the familial genetic duties, especially to impart genetic information to relatives, on the one hand, and the traditional right to individual privacy, on the other. Should a family member be morally obligated to impart such personal information to relatives? Even the law protects the confidentiality of his medical records. The answer involves resolving the conflict by arguing that this right can be justifiably circumscribed. Again, even the law sets limits to this right, when the individual's medical condition affects the public health. (See the paper by Green and Capron in this series for a further elaboration of this point.) In the case at hand, an argument may be plausibly mounted on the basis that an individual's genetic make-up may impinge on the welfare of other family members and is not therefore purely personal in character.

The parent-citizen model of genetic responsibility may be appraised as being reasonably coherent. The main internal problem of this model involves specifying the meaning of the "public interest" or the "public welfare," a problem which is the bane of political philosophy. The traditional controversy only compounds the problem of ascertaining when appeals to the public interest and welfare are really sensible and legitimate. The debate over whether genetic diseases constitute a public health concern signals another important and related issue. These problems cannot be resolved here, but it seems appropriate to suggest that they are not in principle irresolvable. In light of the nature of public interest in genetic disease, namely, the expenditure of public funds and the allocation of scarce medical resources for both research and institutional care, it may be noted that the question of whether economic factors can, or should be, converted into moral considerations is raised by this model also.

A final issue – the conflict between this model's genetic duties and the presumed individual rights to self-determination – should be glaringly obvious. This conflict is well-represented by the development of government-sponsored screening programs, particularly those which prescribe legal sanctions. Although the means of resolving such conflict might be sought in the form mentioned in regard to the other models (namely, by circumscribing individual rights), the argument for such resolution is much less persuasive in this case. This is so for many reasons: First, it is not clear that voluntary screening programs are not sufficient to do the job. Second, the public health nature of genetic disease is still a very debatable matter; thus, the justification for legally sanctioned programs is not at all obvious. Finally, those legally sanctioned genetic screening programs which are being developed do not, in most cases, offer any counseling or therapy; so it is unclear how they benefit the screenees, much less the public as a whole. However, since these objections are contingent in character and resolvable in principle, the potential cogency of the model cannot be ruled out. It must be admitted that the consequences of genetic disease do affect what is called the public interest, both in terms of public funds and the use of the society's medical resources.

Unlike the first three models, *the parent-species member model* of genetic responsibility does not appear to be reasonably coherent. It is replete with internal problems, such as determining what acts are genetically harmful to the species and determining what "accountability to" can sensibly mean in this context. The potential benefits perceived from this model's perspective seem to devolve upon a hoped-for reduction or elimination of seriously defective genes in the human population. Thus, not only is its frame of reference rather vague and indeterminate – the human species as a whole – but its time reference is also vague and indeterminate. As indicated earlier, its principal basis is that acts performed by one generation can significantly affect subsequent generations, but while exploding H-bombs might serve as a paradigm for such acts, it is not clear that procreative acts fall within this category. These unclarities, together with the dubious assumption that serious genetic defects can be reduced or eliminated in the species as a whole, tend to vitiate this model. This judgment, however, does not mean that an amorphous sense of genetic responsibility for the human species is not emerging. Indeed, evidence suggests quite the contrary. Despite its lack of coherence and cogency, this model may still have significant social effects.

Appraising *the parent-ethnic population member model* of genetic responsibility represents a more complex task: it appears that this model may or may not be reasonably coherent, depending upon the case – that is, depending upon which high-risk population is being considered. For example, it may appear reasonably coherent with regard to the black population and sickle cell anemia or the Jewish population and Tay-Sachs disease, but in reference to all women over forty years of age and the Down syndrome, the model looks less plausible. On the whole, this model appears to have many internal problems. The assumption that an ethnic high-risk population forms a large "family" or social community which can serve as the basis for determining duties and rights is a major problem, for community identity and organization may vary widely in degree, even within the same ethnic population. Without a well-defined social basis, the model's articulation of genetic duties which evidently conflict with the recognized rights of voluntary procreation and individual privacy is bound to appear rather arbitrary. The issue of "accountability to" a vague community comprised of many interests and values with no clear consensus or locus of authority highlights the difficulties in this model.

From this very brief discussion of the five models of genetic responsibility, even a provisional assessment of their relative cogency may seem premature. Yet, there is some indication that the parent, family and citizen models may be somewhat more persuasive and viable than the species and ethnic population models. Among these three more cogent models, it appears that the parental and familial models are more persuasive than the citizen model, but this judgment is certainly weaker than the first ranking. Some may view the negative assessment of the ethnic population model as completely off base; however, for the sake of argument, the second part of the appraisal will focus on the three strongest models: the parental, the familial and the citizen.

Appraisal of the Strongest Models

This part of the appraisal will be structured around four central questions raised in concert by these three initially plausible models of genetic responsibility. The questions will serve as an organizational device for elucidating more clearly the sociomoral problems and tensions posed by these three prevalent notions of genetic responsibility. As has been the case throughout this inquiry, the genetic screenee's principal role will be construed as that of a prospective parent. In the following discussion, this role will be approached from the context of the nuclear family, the extended family and civil society: parent simpliciter (nuclear family), parent-family member (extended family) and parent-citizen (civil society). The resulting key questions are these:

1. Do parents have the right to determine, according to their own wishes and notions of what is good for them, the biologic (that is, genetic) quality of their offspring?
2. Do parents have a duty to avoid bearing children with serious genetic defects if this is feasible?
3. Should parents recognize a right on the part of society to intervene in parenthood and shape reproductive behavior?
4. Do parents have a duty to transmit relevant genetic information to relatives that may be at high risk?

The subsequent discussion will take each question one by one and set out supportative considerations for answering the question affirmatively and then countervailing considerations for answering the question negatively.

Do parents have the right to determine, according to their own wishes and notions of what is good for them, the biologic, genetic quality of their offspring? There are three major supportive considerations for answering this question affirmatively. First, it may be argued that the human rights of personal inviolability – the right to life with a self-determined destiny, the right to marry and found a family, the right to voluntary procreation and other rights constitutive of the integrity of the person and of the family – imply freedom of parental choice in reproductive behavior. In short, parents have a right to exercise control over events of major importance to their life-development. Genetic screening and correlated technologies merely enhance this parental freedom by widening parental options and enriching the decision-making process. A second affirmative consideration, obviously related to the first, runs as follows: As part of their role, parents have the right to determine what is in the best interests of their offspring, both actual and potential. Thus acting on their child's behalf, they have the right to decide whether it would be preferable for their child not to be born, particularly if through screening procedures it can be determined that the parents are at high risk for bearing a defective child, or even that the child would most certainly be born with a serious genetic defect. A third affirmative consideration is a bit more involved and needs careful statement. It rests upon the difficulty of assessing the total impact that bearing a genetically defective child would have on a family, including the prospective child itself and other members of the nuclear family. Weighing the significance of disease factors taken by themselves is difficult enough: disease severity, mortality, morbidity, chronic pain, mental retardation, morphologic malformation, etc.; but then assessing the effects of these factors on the prospective child, the parents and other extant children in terms of prolonged distress for the family, or the ability to meet medical costs, complicates the matter many times over. The upshot of indicating the complexities involved in such an assessment is to suggest that perhaps only the parents are, and can be, in a position to weigh these factors and their consequences. In effect, the parents' position may well be unique in this regard; and if this is the case, then perhaps they should be accorded the right to intervene in determining the biologic or genetic quality of prospective progeny insofar as this is possible.

Naturally enough, there are significant countervailing considerations to accepting this parental right. First, it may be argued that the exercise of this parental right, if there be such, conflicts with a fetal right to life. This conflicting fetal right to life, often asserted quite dogmatically, is approached more cautiously by those who point out that as a person in prospect, the fetus cannot argue its own case for being allowed to come to term. As an ironic corollary, the cautious also hold the position that the parents cannot or should not be so "paternalistic" as to think they can properly argue the case on behalf of the fetus for not being brought to term, genetic considerations notwithstanding. A related point, mentioned occasionally but never fully developed, is the view that children, including those in prospect, are not the "property" of parents and therefore are not to be treated as such: this point amounts to a poignant statement of the critique against parental paternalism. A second countervailing consideration is based on the fact that the exercise of the proposed parental right involves an assessment of such factors as the seriousness of a particular genetic disease and thereby invokes such notions as genetic normalcy. The criticisms that are often brought to bear at this point include the following: First, there is an absence, even within the medical profession, of clear-cut definitions and consensuses on what constitutes health, disease, normality and abnormality in general, much less genetic health, genetic disease, genetic normality and genetic abnormality in particular. Apparently, definitions and cutoff points in this area are quite arbitrary, fluctuating and subject to much debate. Moreover, even the severity of a particular genetic disease ranges along a continuum or spectrum of seriousness; indeed, this is the case with most genetic diseases. The thrust of making these observations is to indicate that in the absence of clear-cut definitions in the area of medical genetics, the exercise of the proposed parental right must inevitably appear somewhat arbitrary. Then rhetorical questions such as, "Is it morally justifiable to decide life and death issues on the basis of arbitrary definitions and cutoff points?" are posed in order to argue against the recognition and exercise of the parental right in question. A third and related countervailing consideration addresses directly the uniqueness of the parental position in assessing the significance of genetic factors and their consequences for the nuclear family. It is argued that ascertaining the total impact of a genetic disease, the birth of a genetically defective child, on the child itself and other members of the nuclear family is utterly subjective and relative, being based on arbitrary medical criteria and unconscious preconceptions of what counts as a worthy human being, that is, worthy enough to be allowed to be born. Furthermore, it is pointed out that such parental assessments are notoriously open to change. There are cases in which parents who initially thought they could not bear the burden of rearing a genetically defective child later found hitherto unknown and unpredicted reservoirs of strength adequate to meet the problems. The upshot of this third consideration is an argument to the effect that perhaps parents are not in the best position to make a realistic, objective and dispassionate assessment of all the factors involved in a genetic disease's total impact on the nuclear family.

Do parents have a duty to avoid bearing children with serious genetic defects if this is possible? There are at least three supportive considerations for answering this question in the affirmative. The first and most frequently cited one may be formulated as follows: if the birth and subsequent care of a seriously defective child would probably endanger the welfare of other family members, especially extant children – for example, by drastically reducing their chances for receiving appropriate material support for their basic needs of clothing, medical and dental care, education and the like – then parental rights of self-determination must yield to the more exigent claims of others. A second affirmative consideration involves the increasingly invoked right of every child to be born with a sound mind and healthy body. This right is not only cited by geneticists but also by parents themselves and thus merits serious attention. As suggested earlier in connection with the parental model of genetic responsibility, a more plausible formulation of this right is that every child has a right to be born free of genetic defects and abnormality if this is feasible. The source of this right is not self-evident, but presumably it has something to do with how the basic concepts in the human rights to life and the pursuit of happiness are being defined in terms of a growing consensus on what constitutes an acceptable quality of human life, for example, the capacity for becoming a self-conscious person who can shape his own destiny and fate. If there is such a right, then following the earlier discussion of a correlation between rights and duties, it may be argued that parents have a duty to respect the "exercise" of this right by avoiding, if possible, the birth of children with serious genetic defects. The notion that an unborn child has such a right which can be exercised and must be respected may seem peculiar, but perhaps no more so than the conception of a fetal right to life. In any case, any philosophic perplexity in such matters cannot be resolved here. A third affirmative consideration runs as follows: in a situation of detectable carrier status and available intrauterine diagnosis and selective abortion, for parents to conceive and then intentionally and knowingly bear a genetically defective child would seem to constitute a *prima facie* reckless, inhumane and morally irresponsible course of action, a wrong against the child in question. Although this view is often not developed much beyond this bald charge of immorality, it seems that it can only make sense against the background of the aforementioned child's right; otherwise, the criteria for such a moral evaluation appear lacking.

Countervailing considerations for not recognizing the proposed parental duty principally involve attacking the affirmative considerations. In the first place, it is often pointed out that it is difficult to really calculate and quantify the projected deleterious impact of a defective child on the well-being of a family; again, reminiscent of the second countervailing consideration against the parental right, it is suggested that parents cannot assess objectively the relevant factors involved, that they may have hitherto unknown sources of strength to meet the situation, and so forth. A second countervailing consideration questions the formulation and source of the suggested child's right. It is argued that most formulations of this right employ notions such as sound mind and healthy body which have never been, and perhaps never can be, clearly defined and cogently defended. Moreover, it is claimed that this right sets a biologically unrealistic goal – who can ever ensure that a child will be born with a sound mind and body? The same sort of critique can also be leveled at the more biologically plausible formulation. The notions of genetic health and disease have been handled rather arbitrarily to date. Also, the goal of ensuring that a child be born free of genetic defect is biologically unrealistic: not all genetic conditions, for example, can be detected in utero. If this critique is on target, then it is rhetorically asked, what sense does it make to talk about duties in such matters? A third countervailing consideration is directed against that affirmative consideration involving the charges of virtual malice aforethought and moral blameworthiness. Two points can be brought to bear against such charges: First, it seems rather unjust to "punish" or blame a person for something that is not under his control, as is the fact of being the carrier of a recessive genetic trait. Second and more important, to hold parents morally responsible for the birth of an avoidable defective child, even when they consciously choose to allow such a child to come to term rather than selectively abort it, runs directly counter to parental rights of self-determination and seems to make a sham of the ideal of freedom of parental choice.

Should parents recognize a right on the part of civil society to intervene in parenthood and shape reproductive behavior? This issue is probably the most controversial of the four under investigation. There are at least three supportive considerations for answering the question in the affirmative. All three are related, but for the sake of clarity they will be introduced separately. The first affirmative consideration harks back to the parent-citizen model of genetic responsibility as it was initially developed. It argues that civil society has a legitimate interest in the quality of children to be born in its midst. For example, in order to meet present and future social needs, it should be recognized that society has a stake in maximizing the number of useful people with "social worth" who have the capacity to satisfy such needs. Conversely, society has a stake in minimizing the number of people likely to become public charges and thereby burden society's resources. Thus it may be argued that in order to further the common good, society may, and perhaps should, undertake measures to ensure that each individual, construed as a prospective citizen, is born as healthy as possible and to avoid so far as possible the costs of caring for the genetically defective. One can conceive of a number of possible governmental measures to meet these utilitarian ends; for example, to pose some extremes, mandatory genetic screening and counseling programs, genetic criteria for marriage licenses, genetically indicated fertility controls, negative incentive programs designed to discourage the birth of genetically defective children, etc. A second related affirmative consideration argues that as citizens parents are duty bound to act in the common good; so perhaps they should recognize society's legitimate interest in the biologic quality of progeny and possibly its right to intervene in parenthood and reproduction for the sake of the public interest. The extent of such intervention may be debatable, but it may be argued that intervention in principle has a clear rationale. A third affirmative consideration is yet another variation on the first: if society deems genetic disease to be a public health hazard, then perhaps parents should not only comply with but positively support the suggested forms of genetic intervention on the part of the state.

There are a number of significant countervailing considerations to be taken into account. Four will be mentioned here. First, it needs to be observed that cost-benefit analysis with regard to life and death matters and with reference to judging the social worth of individuals is a notoriously perilous undertaking. How does one quantify in this area and still make moral or even economic sense? Usually such analysis is posed in terms of comparing the costs of preventing the births of defective children with the costs of institutional care. But is it possible to make an accurate economic analysis in this matter? Comparing the long-range costs of extensive governmental intervention against those of institutional care is no easy task. How can one quantify costs such as the erosion of parental freedom and its long-range consequences? Furthermore, judging people in terms of social worth seems to reduce them to a mere nexus of utility functions and overlooks their dignity as persons, a value highly esteemed in our society. A second countervailing consideration goes to the heart of our conception of what a society is all about. Rather than trying to avoid the burden of institutional care and the like, is it not the case that society has an obligation to share the parental burden of caring for defective children? Indeed, is it not incumbent on a humane democratic society to help bear the social costs of exercising individual freedoms? Third, some may argue that making parenthood a matter of privilege is unjust, for in so doing society is infringing on the fundamental human rights of self-determination, liberty, equality, etc. which it has the obligation to protect. Making parenthood a matter of privilege is not merely insensitive – that is not the issue – but rather represents an injustice to the extent that the very basis of what goes to make up a just society is in part eroded: individual freedom, personal inviolability and related human rights lie at the very roots of our society. Finally, as a fourth countervailing consideration that need only be mentioned in passing since it was introduced earlier, it should be clearly underscored that it is quite debatable whether genetic disease does indeed constitute a public health problem. Many geneticists would roundly contest this view of genetic disease. In fact, from a population perspective many geneticists seem to view genetic disease and the presence of deleterious genetic traits as a positive sign of genetic diversity much to be desired, rather than as a negative sign of genetic pollution.

Do parents have a duty to transmit relevant genetic information to relatives in the extended family who may possibly be at high risk for carrying a recessive trait? There are at least two affirmative considerations for recognizing such a duty. First, it should be observed that parents are members of an extended family whose welfare they are committed to or even obligated to serve. The grounds for this commitment and responsibility were introduced in connection with the familial model of genetic responsibility articulated earlier and do not need restatement. Inasmuch as parents are obligated generally to inform other family members of matters relating to their welfare, the duty to transmit relevant genetic information seems to have some warrant. The second affirmative consideration should be obvious; namely, the benefits of transmitting such genetic information may be considerable. Relatives at risk for carrying the recessive trait may become apprised of their carrier status and subsequently exercise their parental rights and duties as informed and responsible agents. Of course, it goes without saying that relatives at risk for expressing the disease condition may seek the necessary medical aid.

There are, however, some countervailing considerations which must be noted. First, it should be observed that recognizing this duty conflicts with the presumed rights to privacy and confidentiality regarding personal medical factors. This conflict may be viewed by some as a legal rather than a moral matter. The release of medical genetic information raises the specter of the possible prejudicial use of genetic information by others, particularly if the information gets beyond the control of the nuclear and extended family. Social stigmatization and discrimination on genetic grounds is a documented social abuse. Finally, without some checks and controls, perhaps by genetic counselors, the parents' transmission of genetic information could create unnecessary and unwarranted concerns and fears in other family members. This latter consideration raises a principally technical issue of how such genetic information should be transmitted, if at all.

Conclusion

The following assessment aims to articulate and defend briefly an acceptable view of genetic responsibility, or what was earlier called a "minimal ethic of genetic responsibility." It seems by far the wisest course to sketch the outlines of this view at the outset, so that suspicions of a hidden agenda are allayed. Briefly stated, the following view will be defended: Parents have the right to determine, according to their own wishes and notions of what is good for them, the genetic quality of their offspring, with the proviso that in certain circumstances they may have the duty to avoid bearing children with serious genetic defects if this is possible. Thus the parental right is not absolute, inasmuch as it is subject to at least one sort of circumscription. Moreover, parents have a duty to permit relevant genetic information to be transmitted to relatives in the extended family if this is medically/genetically indicated. The position here sketched, then, recognizes the validity of selected components of two models of genetic responsibility: the parental model simpliciter and the parent-family member model. And it explicitly rejects the components of the parent-citizen model of genetic responsibility.

A full defense of this position would require the examination of each consideration relating to the four questions explored above. Within the confines of this provisional appraisal, however, it must suffice to identify the prevailing reasons for the position just outlined. All three affirmative considerations in support of recognizing the suggested parental right are eminently plausible, while the countervailing considerations lack validity in the final analysis. The human rights of personal inviolability, self-determination in marrying and founding a family, and voluntary procreation do indeed imply freedom of parental choice in reproductive behavior and the right to determine what is in the best interests of prospective offspring. Moreover, parents are in the best and perhaps unique position to assess the total impact that a genetically defective child may have on themselves and their families, to make realistic predictions of what will contribute to or detract from the welfare and happiness of themselves and their families. Finally, it may be observed that the fetal right to life, if there be such, does not override the parental right for a number of reasons. For example, it may be plausibly argued that a fetus possesses a serious right to life only if it possesses the potentiality to become a self-conscious being capable of self-determination and free agency; this condition is absent in the case of many genetic conditions. Furthermore, it seems plausible to argue that the rights and claims of extant persons are simply more exigent than those ascribed to a person in prospect. Enough said in defense of this parental right, now what about the parental duty circumscribing the exercise of this right?

The position that parents have a duty to avoid, wherever feasible, bearing a child with a serious genetic defect has particular cogency in situations where the birth and subsequent care of such a child would radically endanger the welfare of other family members, especially extant children. Such situations may be viewed as constituting a legitimate circumscription on the exercise of the parental right. The right of parents to undertake the burdens of bearing and caring for a genetically defective child is acknowledged, but when the care of such a prospective child would be likely to affect adversely the welfare of other extant children for whom parents bear a prior responsibility, then perhaps parental wishes, even supererogatory ones, and rights must give way to these more exigent and prior claims.

The question which is raised by recognizing this genetic duty is whether it implies a further duty to be genetically screened. There is no easy answer to this question. But if this is a legitimate duty incumbent on parents in the area of applied human genetics, it seems that any responsible fulfillment of the duty requires some sort of obligation to be genetically screened. The next obvious query is, under what circumstances is there such an obligation? The most plausible and cautious response would seem to be the following: if parents are contemplating the exercise of their right of voluntary procreation, and are at the same time aware that they may be at high risk for bearing a genetically defective child whose birth and care would in their situation endanger the welfare of the nuclear family, then they have the obligation to undergo the relevant available genetic screening procedure.

Before turning to the matter of transmitting genetic information, it should be noted that the countervailing considerations against recognizing a societal right to intervene in parenthood and reproductive behavior seem eminently more persuasive than the utilitarian-based affirmative considerations. The pivotal factor in this negative appraisal is the recognition that the viability of our society rests upon and is designed to protect precisely those fundamental human rights which help to form the basis of the parental role. For our society to encroach upon these rights would be self-defeating and masochistic in the extreme.

The affirmative considerations for recognizing a duty to permit the transmission of genetic information to relatives at high risk far outweigh the negative factors. The duty seems to have a solid moral basis indeed. And the countervailing considerations raise problems which seem more practical and technical in character rather than representing matters of principle. The one possible issue of principle – conflict with a right to privacy – has already been addressed in the initial assessment of the familial model of genetic responsibility. The point made there was that genetic information impinging on the welfare of other family members is by its very nature not merely a matter of purely personal and private concern. A somewhat puzzling question is whether recognizing this genetic duty implies a further duty to be genetically screened. That is, does the obligation to transmit genetic information imply the duty to acquire such information? The puzzling nature of this question can perhaps be elucidated by the following situation: a citizen who happens to see a crime committed has the obligation to report this information to the proper authorities, but it is not at all clear that he has the duty to go around hunting up crimes to report. For this sort of reason, among others, it is not patently clear that the genetic duty to transmit relevant information implies the duty to acquire such information by undergoing genetic screening.

Much more could be said by way of developing and justifying this conception of genetic responsibility. However, these brief concluding remarks are intended only to suggest certain minimally acceptable elements of genetic responsibility which many might agree are valid points of orientation to the issue. These proposals are made in the spirit of trying to crystallize some moral values in this area of medical genetics where so many different moral points of view are brought to bear by genetic screenees and genetic counselors alike.

References

1. Research Group on Ethical, Social and Legal Issues in Genetic Counseling and Genetic Engineering of the Institute of Society, Ethics and the Life Sciences: Ethical and social issues in screening for genetic disease. *New Eng. J. Med., 286*:1129-1132, 1972.
2. Downie, R. S.: *Roles and Values.* London:Methuen & Co. Ltd., 1971.
3. Hart, H. L. A.: *Punishment and Responsibility.* New York:Oxford University Press, 1968.
4. Benn, S. I. and Peters, R. S.: *The Principles of Political Thought.* New York:The Free Press, 1965.
5. Callahan, D.: *Abortion: Law, Choice and Morality.* New York:The Macmillan Publishing Company, 1970.
6. Adams, D. N.: *The American Family.* Chicago:Markham Publishing Co., 1971.
7. Fletcher, J.: The brink: The parent-child bond in the genetic revolution. *Theological Studies, 33*:457-485.
8. Motulsky, A.: The significance of genetic disease. In Hilton, B. et al (eds.) *Ethical Issues in Human Genetics.* New York:Plenum Press, 1973.
9. Fraser, F. C.: Survey of counseling practices. In Hilton, B. et al (eds.): *Ethical Issues in Human Genetics.* New York:Plenum Press, 1973.
10. Crow, J. F.: Population perspective. In Hilton, B. et al (eds.): *Ethical Issues in Human Genetics.* New York:Plenum Press, 1973.

Subject Index

SUBJECT INDEX